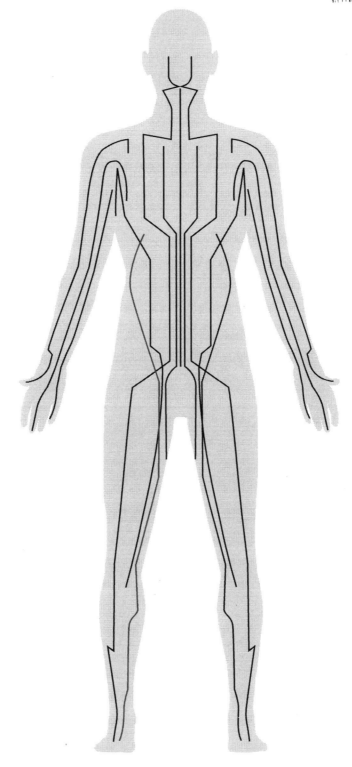

Treat Yourself with Acupressure

Adriana Germain

An easy way to relieve pain, tension, anxiety and stress.
Gain vibrant health and look years younger.

Cover Design & Graphic Production – English Edition
Johanna Leovey

The publisher is grateful to the following copyright holders
for permission to reproduce the following materials:

Photography
Pete Aarre-Ahtio 2003
from Parantavat pisteet.
Hoida itseasi akupainannalla.

Illustrations
Marienka Pakaslahti 2003
from Parantavat pisteet.
Hoida itseasi akupainannalla.

ISBN 978-0-615-42180-3
English Edition, 2010

First published in Finland in 2003 as *Parantavat pisteet.*
*Hoida itseasi akupainannall*a.

PRINTED IN THE UNITED STATES

The tchniques, ideas, and suggestions in this book are not intended as a substitute for proper medical advice.
Any application of the techniques, ideas, and suggestions in this book is at the reader's sole discretion and risk.

Contents

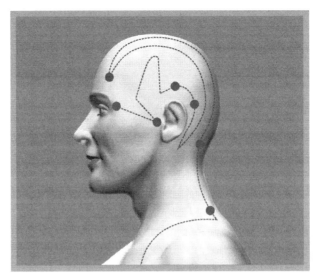

Introduction

What is acupressure?

Thousands of years ago the Chinese learned that pressing certain points on the skin one could induce favorable effects somewhere else in the body. That is acupressure.

Acupressure is based on the Chinese concept of qi, the basic energy of the universe. Qi regulates all the vital functions of the human body: the beating of the heart, the breath, the birth and the decay of the cells, the sexuality and the emotions. Man stays healthy as long as there is enough qi, and it flows freely. One becomes ill if qi starts to decrease or gets stuck.

Pressing the acupressure points in the body can augment qi. It releases stagnations, and the energy is free to flow. Every acupressure point is named according to its function:

"The Gate of Wind" treats the flu and aches, while "The Sea of Blood" treats menstrual problems. In the West, however, the points are called more practically according to their numbers.

The acupressure points are located along twelve energy meridians. These meridians, invisible to the eye, are channels along which the qi flows in the body. One can access the qi of the meridians by inserting ultra thin needles in them or by pressing them with fingers. Acupressure is a method for self-help and is suitable for those who do not like the idea of needles inserted into the skin.

Many illnesses need the intervention of modern Western medicine. But knowing the basic anatomy of the body and following the descriptions of this book, it is easy to learn to alleviate the pain and swelling, to improve the blood circulation, and to activate the metabolism. Acupressure also works well as a preventive treatment because it improves the immune system and releases stress.

Acupressure is an excellent method for treating friends and family. It does not need any preparations and can be done fully clothed. Therefore, it can be used also in the workplace, in front of a coffee table or a computer.

How does it work?

The human body is like a large electromagnetic field where acupuncture meridians work as electrical conductors carrying messages to the brain. The brain responds by sending back the appropriate level of direct current to stimulate the healing of the troubled area. Because any current grows weaker with distance, the acupressure points work like little booster amplifiers to get the signal back up to strength while traveling along the meridian.

When the acupressure points are treated with metal needles, electricity or fingers, the brain also releases endorphins, the body's natural opiates, which block the pain, calm the heart, lower the blood pressure and relax the muscles. That improves the blood and lymph circulation, the cells get more oxygen and the swelling disappears.

The whole autonomic nervous system calms down. As a result the immune system gets stronger and prevents us from falling sick.

Touch and pressure are very old and intuitive healing methods. When a child gets hurt in his knee, his mother's hand placed on the knee is enough to stop the pain. When a man hits his toe on a stone, he instinctively grabs it with his hand and presses hard. Pressure feels good.

The entire surface of the body is an interlocking mosaic of dermatomes. Dermatomes are areas of skin supplied with nerves from one spinal root. Loss of sensation of a dermatome signifies damage to a particular nerve root in the spine: Numbness of some fingers might signify a problem in a cervical vertebra, while sciatic pain might be about a herniated disc in the lower back.

The nerves of the skin are connected to the internal organs by the central nervous system. This connection can be used both to detect and to treat ailments inside the body.

What is it used for?

Acupressure can be used to treat many ailments. It alleviates stress and treats sports injuries. It firms and relaxes muscles and activates blood and lymph circulation.

It can also be helpful for many skin conditions, such as acne, eczema, wrinkles, and dry and worn-out skin. Pressure on the acupressure points tones the facial nerves and makes the skin look younger and healthier.

Acupressure is an efficient method to treat back, neck and shoulder pain, stiffness and numbness, headache and migraine, insomnia, depression and panic attacks, cramps, sciatica, menstrual and menopausal problems, asthma and high blood pressure.

When the symptoms disappear, one must still treat the cause. Sometimes it can be done by acupressure alone; sometimes one needs the help of modern Western medicine. Even then, acupressure is a good complementary treatment. Acupuncture and acupressure are routinely used in China in the rehabilitation of paralyzed patients.

One might wonder how one point can have several, very different uses. The point Liver 3, for example, can treat headache, menstrual problems, eye problems, depression and acne. That is because one single point does not alone cure the sickness, but the same point combined with different other points can have different health effects.

It often happens that by pressing on some points to treat a certain illness, another ailment is also cured. Treat flu and fever by pressing Large Intestine 11, and constipation also will be cured.

How to locate the acupressure points

According to traditional Chinese medicine, there are almost five hundred acupressure points in the human body. For the beginner, it is sufficient to know only the most important of them. You find them by following the bones, muscles and other anatomical landmarks. Remember also the Chinese saying "where the pain, there the point".

At first locating the point might feel difficult. You might need to press a large area of the skin before you find the right spot. It always feels slightly sore and different than the surrounding tissue. That's why it is easier to locate a point on your own body than on somebody else.

Ask for feedback when locating the points on another person. The person you are treating can usually sense when your finger is pressing the right point. Practice helps. When you get a bit more experience, your fingers start to automatically detect the right point. It often feels colder and harder than the surrounding area, and it trembles slightly. You learn to recognize these very slight sensations.

To locate the point within half an inch of exactitude is sufficient. When you read "press point Lung 2" in the text, it means that you must press the point number 2 in the Lung meridian. See the chapter on Meridians and Acupressure points starting on page 125.

How to press the acupressure points

Press with a thumb, finger, knuckle, fist, or even with a blunt stick directly on the point. Start with a light pressure and penetrate gradually deeper into the muscle. Hold a steady and continuous pressure approximately for a minute. All your movements must be slow, calm and even, never brusque or sudden. Do not massage except when specifically mentioned in the text.

Sometimes it is better to hold the pressure even longer, until the pain disappears. The pain often radiates to the forehead, when you press the points in the neck. Hold the pressure as long as the pain gradually begins to vanish.

Often the treatment you give to another person has better results than when you treat yourself. It is because you are careful not to induce pain to yourself and do not press hard enough. Some pain is a normal reaction when pressing a tense muscle. When the tension is relieved, the pain disappears.

It is obvious, however, that you should not penetrate a hard muscle too deep immediately. Start with light pressure the first day and go deeper only in the following days.

Always ask for feedback when you treat someone. People are different. Some like or even require the application of very hard pressure, while others prefer a lighter touch. Also, give feedback yourself, when treated by someone else. Tell him or her how the treatment feels. Acupressure must be pleasant, not just tolerable.

Press the points on both sides of the body. Exceptions are some clearly local problems, like tennis elbow and carpal tunnel syndrome. Even then, it is good to press the inflammation point Large Intestine 11 on both sides of the body.

For maximum benefit, acupressure should be done every day. Twice a day is even better. You do not have to press all the points every time: it is sufficient if you choose some of them.

Lots of toxins are released from the body during the treatment, and it is important to drink a lot of water afterward. Also take a rest and dress warmly, as acupressure lowers blood pressure and the body temperature.

Acupressure and psychosomatic illnesses

Traditional Chinese medicine sees the mind and body as a whole and understands the connection between the mind and somatic illnesses.

When a traditional Chinese doctor sees the patient for the first time, the doctor always asks him what happened in his life on the outset of the illness. Was there a change in his living conditions? Did he start a new job or were there problems in the old one? Did he get married or divorced?

Because emotional balance is so important for the physical health, the "seven emotions" are considered as a major cause of illness in traditional Chinese medicine. Although anger, sadness, fear and worry are perfectly normal emotions, they can sometimes overwhelm the body's adaptation mechanism and the person falls ill. It is said in traditional Chinese medicine that sorrow damages the heart, fear damages the lungs, and anger damages the liver.

The Chinese understood early on that when the organs and the muscles do not function properly, there cannot be harmony in the mind. A healthy body is important for a healthy mind. Acupressure is an excellent method for balancing both the mind and the body. The touch calms the body and relaxes the mind. It also creates a strong connection to the environment.

When a nurse is taking a patient's pulse, his heart starts beating regularly, even if it had been irregular before that. It has also been proven that the power of touch enhances the immune system and is the best medicine for depression.

Is acupressure safe?

Acupressure is a perfectly safe method and does not cause any side effects. Acupressure is done by fingertips and anyone can learn it easily. It does not do any harm even if you do not find exactly the right point or even if you press a wrong point by accident.

Acupressure balances the energy of the body and brings the body to a condition of proper functioning. That is why you can use the same point to slow down and to activate an organ. The pressure and the number of the points must, however, be adapted to each person's physical condition. An old and weak person should naturally be treated more lightly than a young and healthy one. The pressure must feel good and slightly painful at the same time.

Some areas of the body are especially sensitive. Use a light pressure while treating the stomach area, and do not press at all on the stomach points if there is a reason to suspect some interior disease. A pregnant woman should not be pressed on points of the stomach, lower back and sacrum, or the point Large Intestine 4 (between the thumb and the forefinger), Spleen 6 (beside the shinbone), Bladder 60 (on the calf), and Bladder 67 (on the little toe).

Also, be careful when you press the body areas with lots of lymph nodes, like the groin and the neck. In addition, do not press inflamed, burned or otherwise damaged skin, or close to a recent operation scar. You can, however, press the area around it. That stimulates the blood circulation, alleviates the swelling, and accelerates the healing.

Treatments For Common Illnesses

Anxiety and Depression

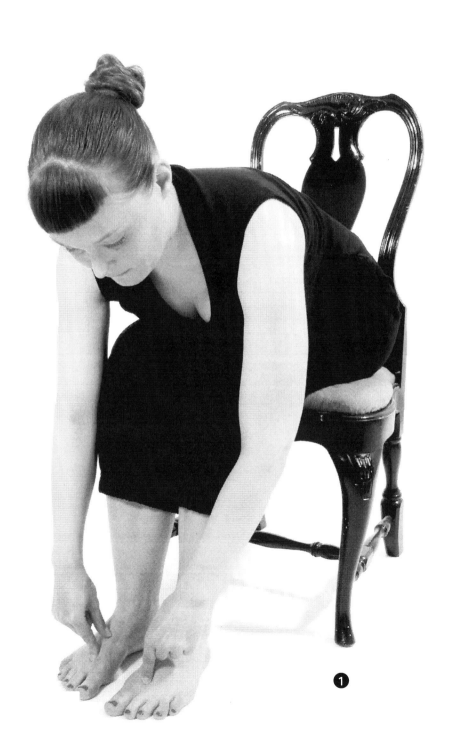

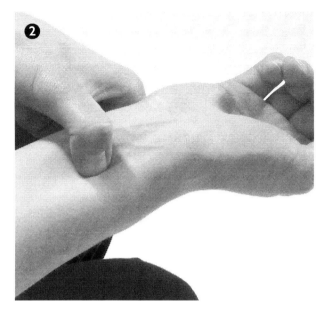

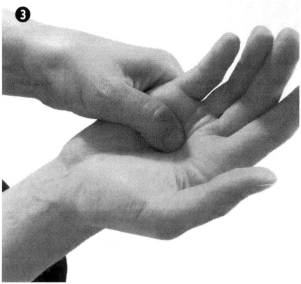

According to traditional Chinese medicine, the internal organs control the emotions. Depression, anxiety and anger can be signs of an improper liver or lung functioning. That works also the other way around: depression and anxiety damage the lungs. When our mood is down, we slump our backs, which makes the breathing shallow. When we do not get enough oxygen, we start sighing and gasping. This is a sign that the lungs do not function at their maximum capacity.

Thus, the basic points to treat depression and anxiety are the liver and lung points. Try to press them several times a day.

It is also important for you to circulate your energy by physical movement. Walking is enough, but it should be done for two hours a day. Increase your energy by eating at least one warm meal a day.

1. Sit on a chair and place your thumbs on the top of your feet in the depression between the big and the second toe. This point is Liver 3, the basic point against depression and stress. Hold a firm and steady pressure, even if the point feels very tender. Press this point on both feet.

2. Press with your thumb on the point Pericardium 6 on the wrist of the other hand. It is located in the middle of the inner side of the forearm, two thumb widths from the wrist crease. Hold a firm pressure between the big tendons. This is the point that calms the mind.

3. Find the point Pericardium 8 in the middle of your palm. You will find it by bending your fingers until the tip of the middle finger touches the palm. The Pericardium 6 point is located here. Press on the point with the thumb of the other hand.

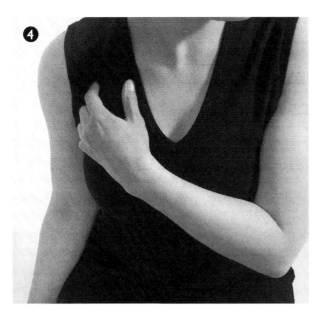

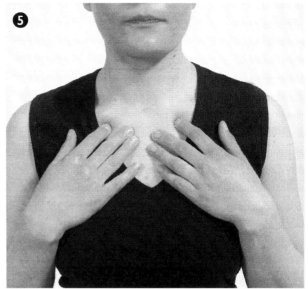

4. Slide your forefinger right under the collarbone along the muscle toward the shoulder. The Lung 2 point is located in a small depression in the outer portion of the chest muscle just before the shoulder. It is often very tender. After locating Lung 2, do not press it. You are going to use Lung 2 in order to find the Lung 1 point, which is three fingers' width directly below Lung 2 and is also tender. Press on Lung 1 with your fingers. Follow this procedure on both sides of your chest in order to press both of the Lung 1 points.

5. Slide your forefingers along the muscle right below the collarbone toward the breastbone. The point Kidney 27 is located in the depression below the collarbone right next to the breastbone. Press the points on both sides of the breastbone with your forefingers.

6. Find a tender spot in the middle of the breastbone, at the level of the nipples. Press the point Ren 17 firmly with a fingertip.

7. Make a loose fist with both hands and rub your back with circular movements from the waist up. On both sides of the spine, in the middle of the long back muscles or latissimus dorsae, about one palm's width upward from the waist is located an important energy point, Bladder 23. Rub this point vigorously in the morning and during the day.

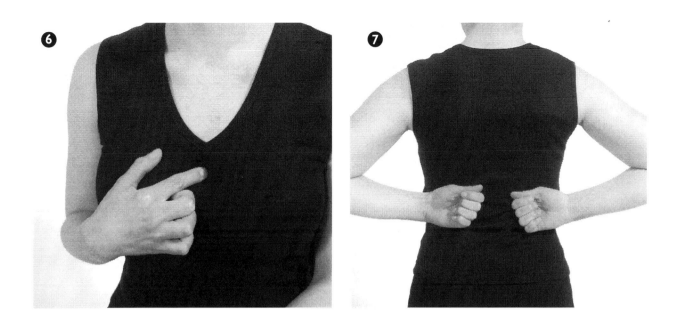

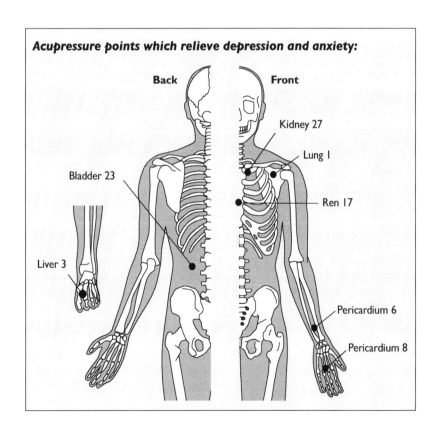

Acupressure points which relieve depression and anxiety:

Back   Front

Kidney 27

Lung 1

Bladder 23

Ren 17

Liver 3

Pericardium 6

Pericardium 8

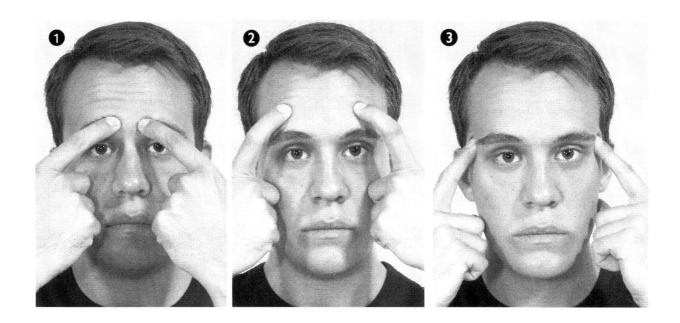

Bell's Palsy

Bell's Palsy is an inflammation of the facial nerve which can happen overnight. For example, going to sleep under a fan or in front of an open window on a hot summer night can paralyse the muscles of the face so that one side of the face starts drooping. One has difficulty in closing one eye, frowning with the forehead and smiling with both sides of the mouth. Usually Bell's palsy goes away in a few weeks. Sometimes, however, one side of the face stays permanently paralyzed.

In China, Bell's palsy is treated by acupuncture. The treatment is first done every other day, then with less frequency. The patient is also advised to press the following acupressure points twice a day.

1. Place your fingers on the inner or medial extremity of the eyebrow. The point Bladder 2 is located on the upper corner of the eye socket. Press up toward the bone. It is easier to press if you tilt your head down and let it relax onto your forefingers.

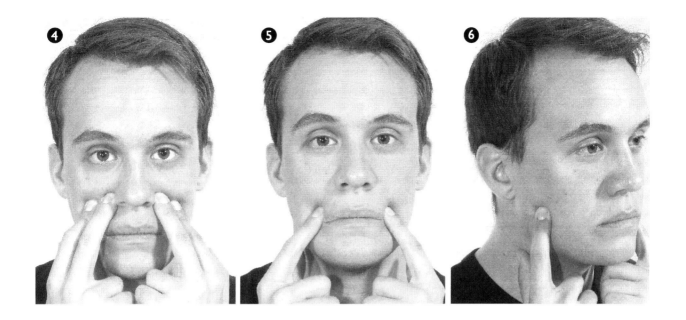

2. At one thumb's width directly above the middle point of the eyebrow, in a direct vertical line with the pupil, you'll find a small depression in the frontal bone. Feel a tender spot on the bone. This is the point Gallbladder 14. Press on the point.

3. Use your forefingers to gently press on your temples. This point is Taiyang.

4. Place your middle and index fingers beside your nostrils underneath the cheekbones. There you will find the points Large Intestine 20 and Stomach 3. Press up toward the bone.

5. Place your forefingers beside the corners of your mouth, directly below the centers of the eyes. Press on the two points called Stomach 4.

6. Move your forefingers to the corners of the jaw-bone and press with a firm pressure on the points Stomach 6.

Also press on the following points: Gallbladder 20 and Large Intestine 4. You'll find their location in the chapter Flu (p. 36).

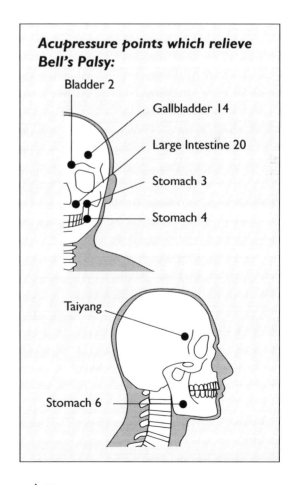

Acupressure points which relieve Bell's Palsy:

Bladder 2

Gallbladder 14

Large Intestine 20

Stomach 3

Stomach 4

Taiyang

Stomach 6

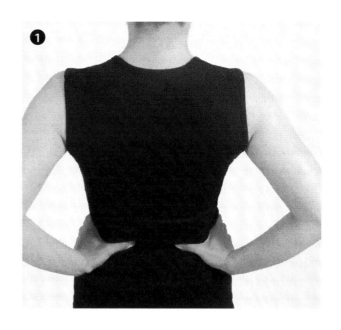

Constipation

Acupressure relaxes the stomach muscles and encourages bowel movements. But it is also important to keep your whole body moving, eat lots of fiber and drink enough water. Elderly people are not likely to drink enough water – the feeling of thirst diminishes with age – it is good to measure eight glasses of water in a jug in the morning and drink it gradually during the day. If you are badly constipated, begin your morning by drinking one glass of warm prune juice. Add a handful of coarse salt to the bathwater, lie down in the tub with your knees up, and rub your stomach thoroughly with your fist with circular motions around the belly button.

Acupressure is most helpful if done several times a day. You do not have to press all the points every time.

1. Rub your lower back and sacrum with loose fists, making circular motions. Place your hands at the waist and press with your thumbs in the middle of the long back muscles on the point Bladder 25. Then rub your stomach with a fist clockwise around the belly button. Do not just rub the skin but press deep into the stomach muscle.

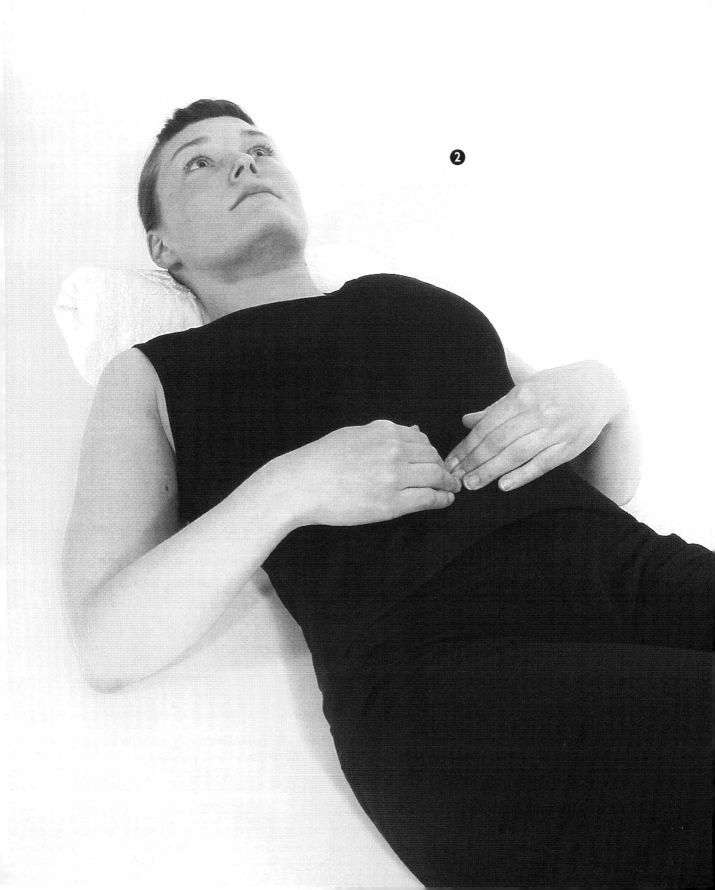

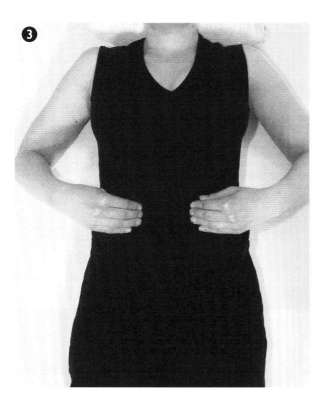

2. Lie down on your back and bend your knees. Place your fingertips or your fist halfway between the base of the breastbone and the belly button. This is the point Ren 12, an important acupressure point for digestion. Press on the point gently. (See previous page.)

3. Place your hands on both sides of the belly button. The points Stomach 25 are located on both sides and two fingers' width from the belly button, in the stomach muscle. Press gently at first, and then gradually increase the depth of the pressure.

4. Place your fingertips two fingers' width below the belly button. This is the location of the point Ren 6. Press gently at first, and then gradually increase the pressure. Hold the pressure for several minutes and breathe deeply.

5. Press with your thumb in the web between the thumb and the forefinger on the back of your hand. This point is Large Intestine 4. Press toward the bone that connects with your index finger.

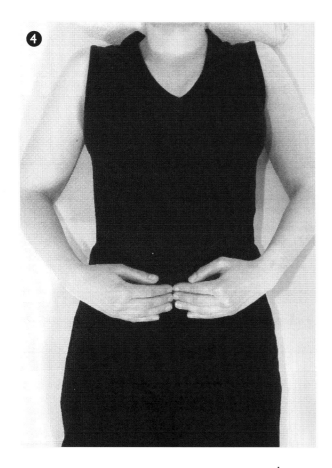

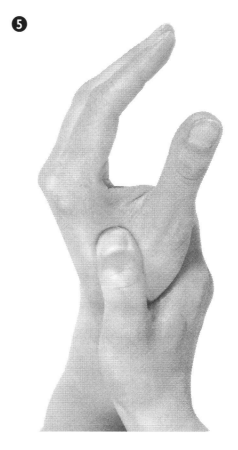

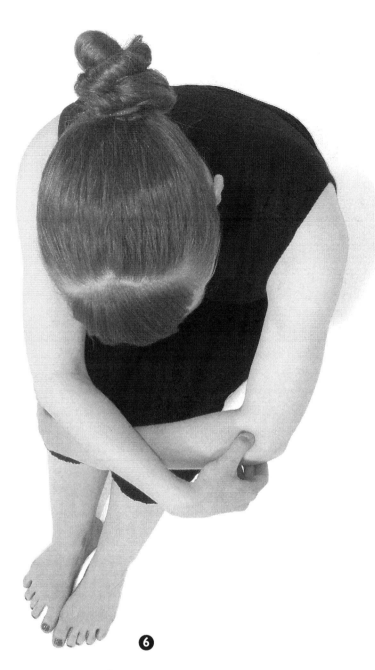

6

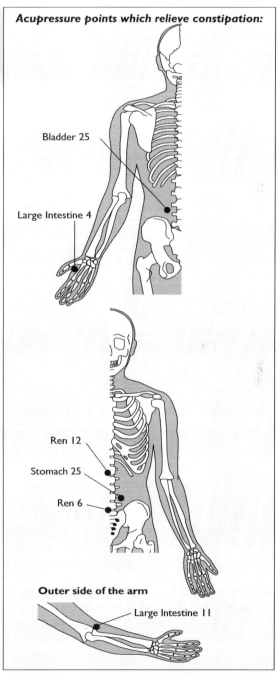

Acupressure points which relieve constipation:

Bladder 25

Large Intestine 4

Ren 12

Stomach 25

Ren 6

Outer side of the arm

Large Intestine 11

6. Bend your elbow. Press with your thumb at the end of the elbow crease on the outside of your forearm on the point Large Intestine 11.

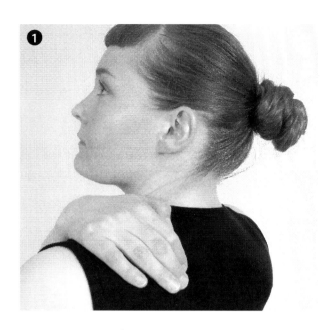

Cough and Asthma

Asthma is treated in traditional Chinese medicine preventatively. The treatments start for months before the season the attacks usually occur, continue during the attacks and several weeks after the symptoms subside. During an attack, and even before it, pain will be felt when the acupressure points of the lung are pressed.

Sit on a chair and breathe deep when pressing the points. When you feel phlegm rising from your lungs, do not swallow it, but spit it out.

You do not have to press all the points every time. You can choose for instance Lung 1 and 2 and press them several times of day or when you feel difficulties in breathing. You'll notice immediate improvement. Remember to press the points on both sides of the body.

1. Bend your right hand over your left shoulder and press with your fore or middle finger halfway between the shoulder blade and the spine below the third thoracic vertebra. This is point Bladder 13, an important point for the lungs. Hold a deep, steady pressure and take long, deep breaths.

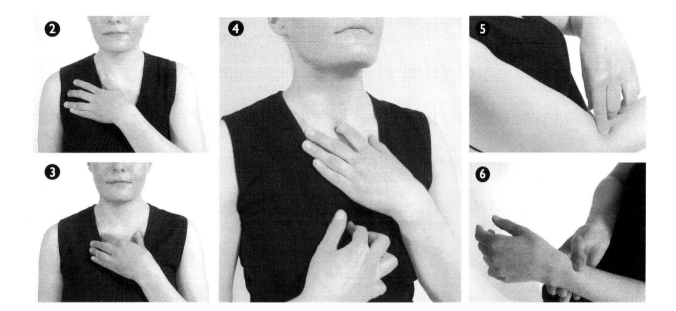

2. Slide your forefingers along the muscle below the collarbone toward the shoulders. Point Lung 2 is located in a depression in the outer portion of the chest muscle just before the shoulder joint. Find the sensitive point below the end of the collarbone. Three fingers' width directly below Lung 2 is another tender point, Lung 1. You may find both points by pressing the outer portion of the chest muscle firmly with your fingers until you find sensitive points below your collarbone. Press both points simultaneously with your middle and forefingers.

3. Slide your forefingers along the muscle right below the collarbone toward the breastbone. The point Kidney 27 is located in the depression below the collarbone right next to the breastbone. Press the points on both sides of the breastbone with your thumb and forefinger.

4. Find a tender spot in the middle of the breastbone, at the level of the nipples. Press the point Ren 17 firmly with the fingertips of one hand. Use the forefinger of the other hand to press in the depression immediately above the breastbone. Use here a very light pressure and a downward angle.

5. Bend your elbow. In the groove of the elbow, on the outer side of the big tendon you'll find the point Lung 5. Press on the point with a firm pressure.

6. Press with your thumb on the point Lung 7. It is located on the arm bone, one inch upward from the wrist.

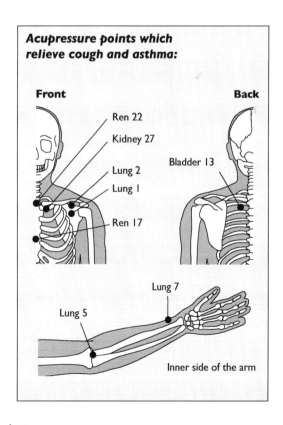

Acupressure points which relieve cough and asthma:

Front

Ren 22
Kidney 27
Lung 2
Lung I
Ren 17

Back

Bladder 13

Lung 7
Lung 5

Inner side of the arm

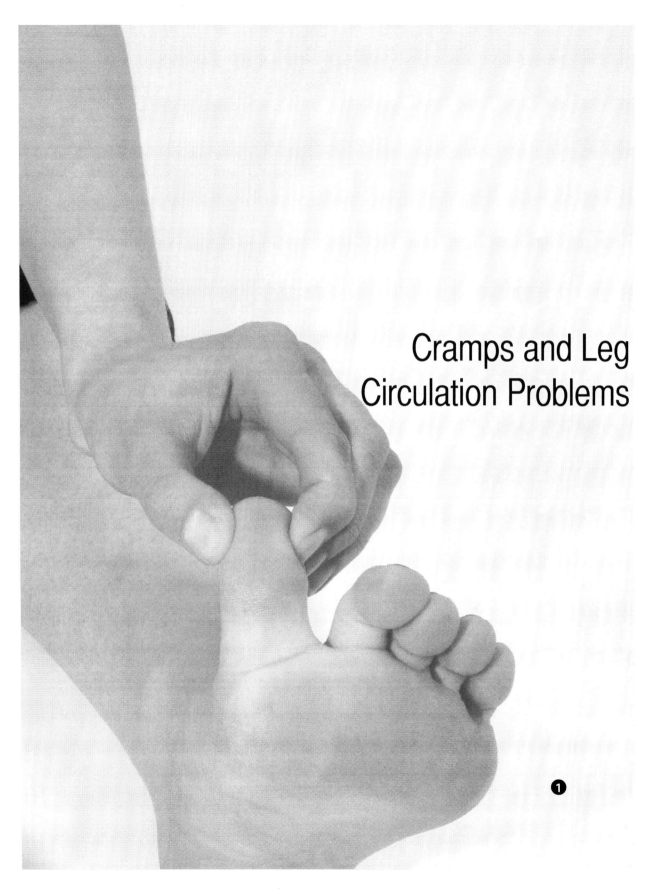

Cramps and Leg Circulation Problems

❷

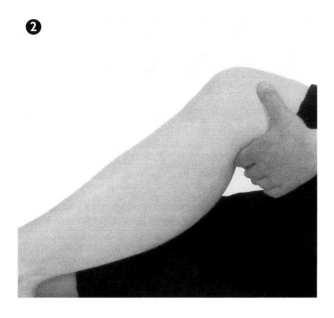

❸ **❹**

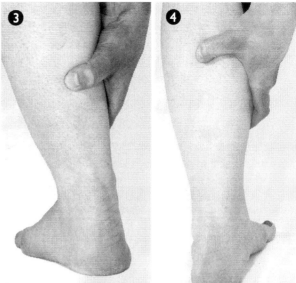

The most common cause for leg cramps is overuse, vigorous exercise or lack of oxygen in the muscles because of cold weather and poor blood circulation. Cramps at nighttime, such as "charley horses," might also be a sign of lack of calcium or magnesium in the body. Try adding minerals in the food or taking mineral supplements to see if the cramps disappear.

Acupressure prevents and relieves the cramps by relaxing the calf muscles. It also improves the blood circulation so that the cells get more oxygen.

1. First rub the calf vigorously. Then grab the big toe and pull it several times toward yourself.

2. Press on the point Bladder 40 in the center of the groove behind the knee. Use a gentle pressure.

3. Place your fingers at the point where the calf muscle bulge joins the Achilles tendon. Keep pressing around the area until you find a tender point. This is Bladder 57. Press on the point firmly.
Diagrams on following page:

4. Press in the middle of the calf muscle on the point Bladder 56. It is the highest point of the calf when the leg is outstretched.

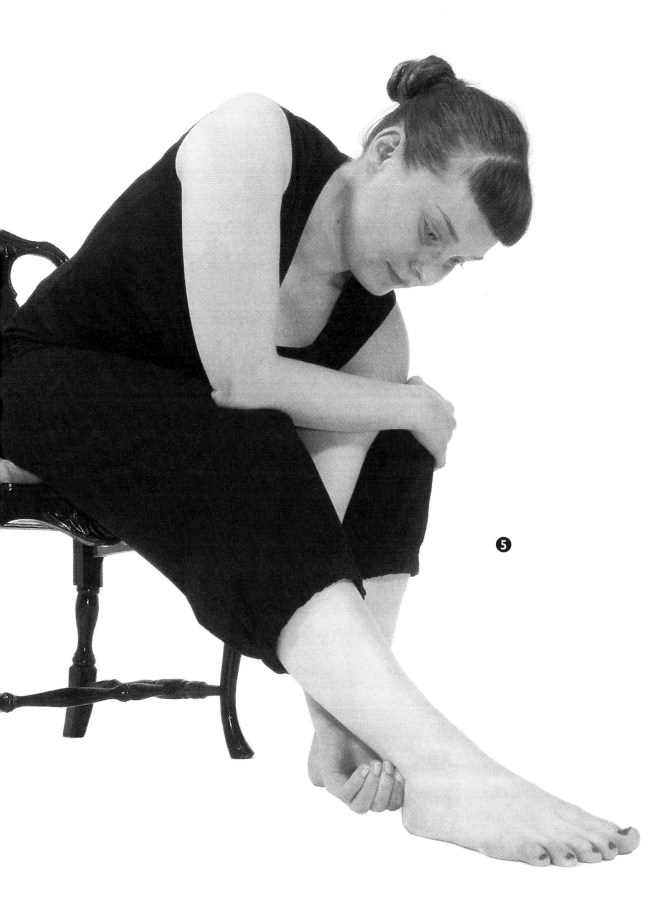

❺

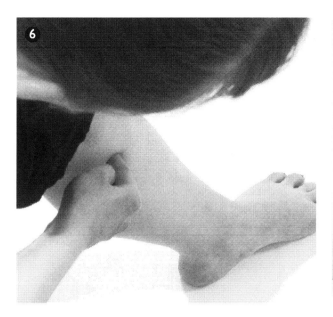

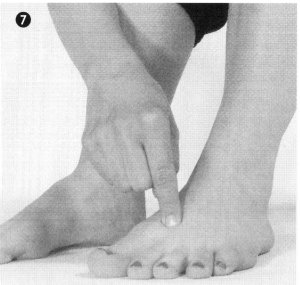

5. Place your thumb on the point Kidney 3 on the inner side of the ankle, in the hollow between the internal malleolus and the Achilles tendon. Place your forefinger on the point Bladder 60 on the outside of the ankle, in the hollow between the external malleolus and the Achilles tendon. Firmly press both points toward each other.

6. On the inner side of the leg there is a big bony lump below the knee. This is the head of the shinbone. Spleen 9 is located below the bone. Press on the point.

7. Place your thumb on top of each foot in the depression between the big toe and the second toe. This point is Liver 3. Hold a firm and steady pressure.

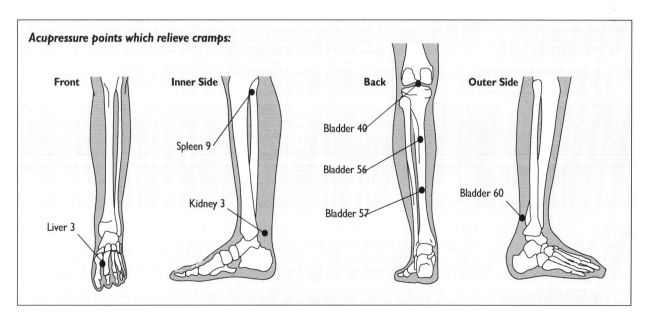

Acupressure points which relieve cramps:

Front   **Inner Side**   **Back**   **Outer Side**

Spleen 9

Kidney 3

Liver 3

Bladder 40

Bladder 56

Bladder 57

Bladder 60

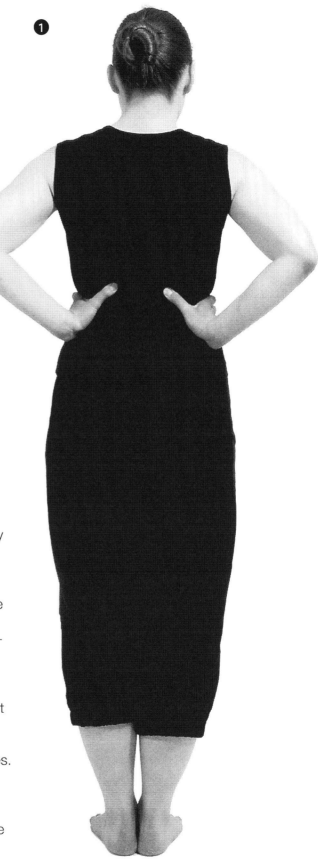

Diarrhea

The cause of sudden diarrhea is often a minor food poisoning, which will usually improve quickly and heal itself in a couple of days. Chronic diarrhea, however, might be a symptom of an illness of an internal organ, and it is better to consult a doctor to find out the cause of it. Often the cause of the diarrhea is not found, since the problem can be caused by diet, eating habits or an irregular lifestyle of the patient. The digestive system is the first to react to psychological stress. Stress is often the cause of irritable bowel syndrome, in which diarrhea and constipation alternate in short succession.

Daily acupressure can calm and balance the digestive system and tone the abdominal muscles. Here is what to do:
Rub, with your fists, the lower back, waist, and sacrum with circular movements. Then press with the thumbs the long, tight muscles along the spine.

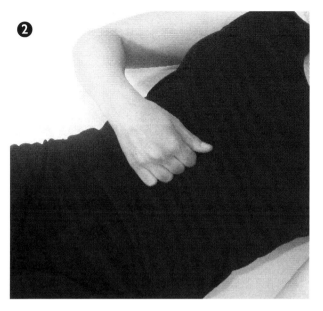

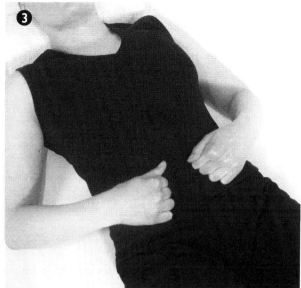

1. Place both hands on the waist. On either side of the spine, one hand's width above the waist, in the middle of the long back muscle, is located the point Bladder 23. Press on the point with your thumbs.

2. Lie down on your back and bend your knees. Place your fingertips or a fist on halfway between the base of the breastbone and the belly bottom. This is Ren 12, an important point for digestion. Press on the point lightly.

3. Place your fingertips on both sides of the belly button. The point Stomach 25 is located two fingers' width from the belly button, in the middle of straight stomach muscle. Press lightly at first, gradually increasing the depth of the pressure.

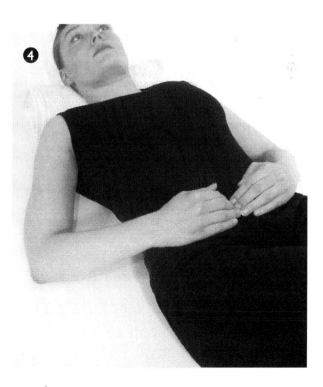

4. Place your fingertips at two fingers' width below the belly button. This is the point Ren 6. Press lightly at first, gradually increasing the pressure. Hold the pressure for several minutes and breathe deeply.

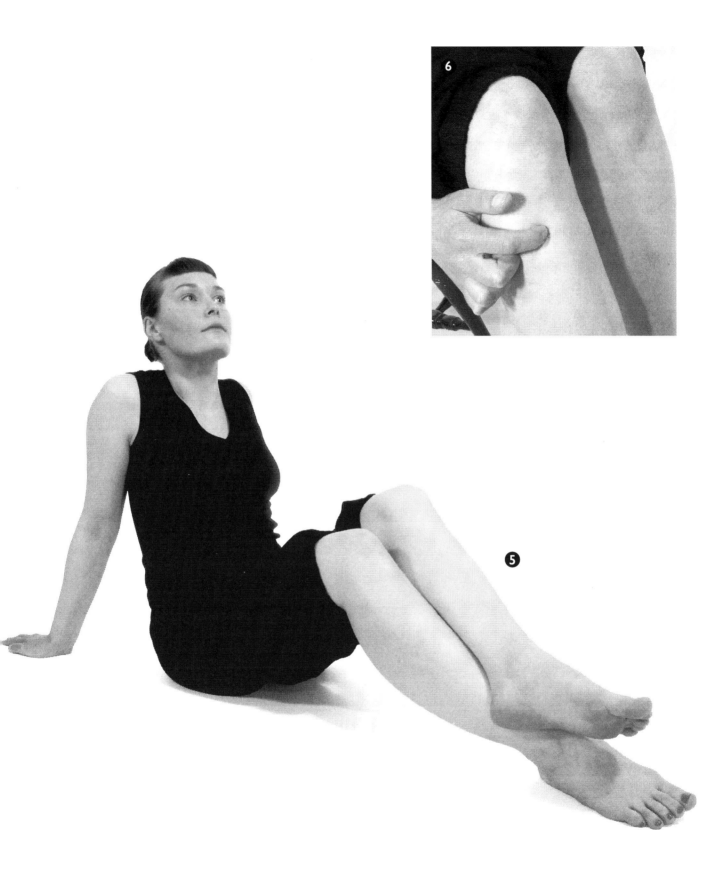

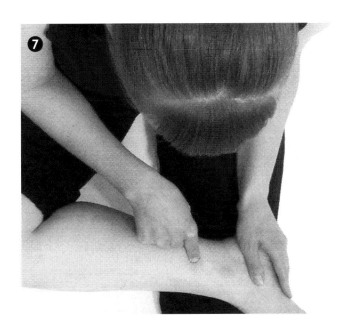

7

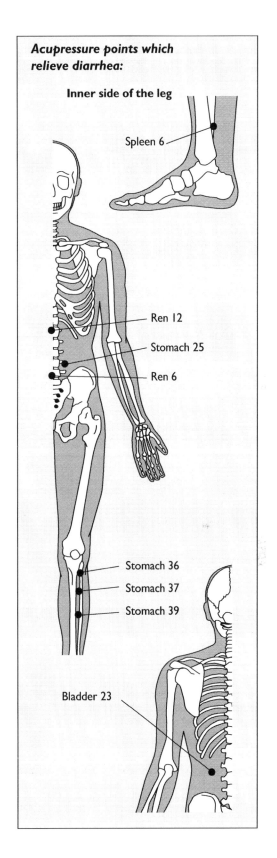

Acupressure points which relieve diarrhea:

Inner side of the leg

Spleen 6

Ren 12

Stomach 25

Ren 6

Stomach 36

Stomach 37

Stomach 39

Bladder 23

5. Sit on the floor and place your right heel on your left leg. Rub with your heel up and down along the outside of the shinbone. When rubbing the area, you stimulate the Stomach meridian and the important digestion points Stomach 36, 37 and 39.

6. You can also press the Stomach meridian points one by one: Stomach 36 is located four fingers' width below the kneecap, one finger width on the outside of the shinbone. Stomach 37 is four fingers' width below Stomach 36, and Stomach 39 is four fingers' width below Stomach 37. All the points are at one finger width on the outside or lateral side of the shinbone.

7. Press on the point Spleen 6. It is located on the inner side of the ankle, at four fingers' width above the internal malleolus, between the shinbone and the Achilles tendon. Find a tender spot in the muscle very close to the bone, but not on it.

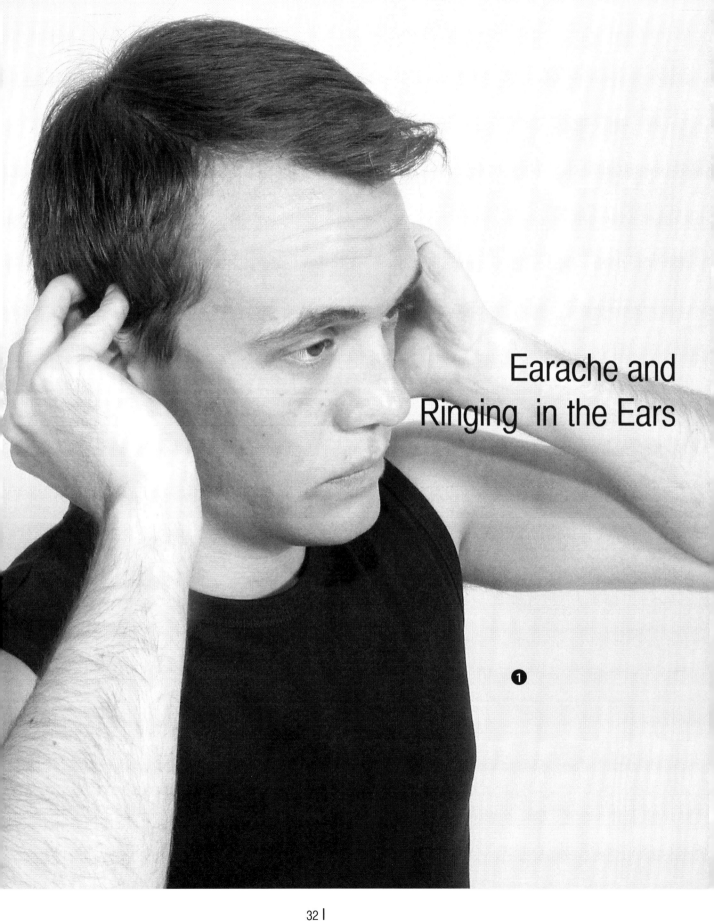

Earache and
Ringing in the Ears

❶

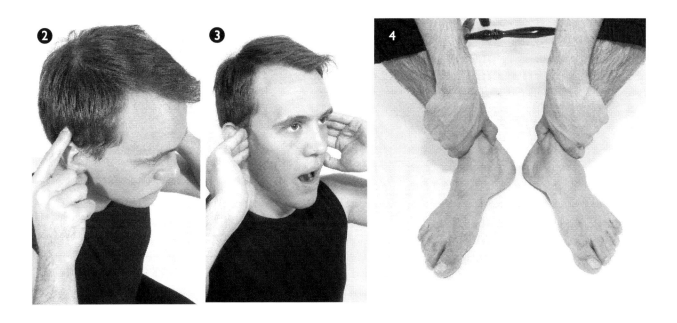

Acupressure relieves the earache caused by wind, cold and changes in air pressure. It also helps to reduce the ringing in the ears. An acute ear infection, however, needs the care of a physician. But even during the medical care it is profitable to press the acupressure points, as it makes the healing faster.

1. Rub your skull vigorously behind the ears. Start the rubbing from the hairline above the ear and progress toward the base of the skull. Repeat three times.

2. Place your forefinger on the point Triple Warmer 20 just above the ear, and your thumb on the point Triple Warmer 17 in the depression under the ear and between the ear and the jawbone. Press both of the points.

3. Open your mouth and place your fore-, middle- and ring fingers in front of the ear hole, in the deep and narrow indentation between the chin- and the skull bone. Press on the points Triple Warmer 21, Small Intestine 19 and Gallbladder 2. Close your eyes and hold the pressure for a couple of minutes.

4. Press on the point Kidney 3 in the rear part of the inside of the ankle, in the hollow between the internal malleolus and the Achilles tendon.

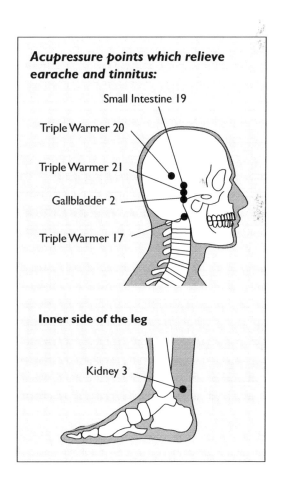

Acupressure points which relieve earache and tinnitus:

Small Intestine 19

Triple Warmer 20

Triple Warmer 21

Gallbladder 2

Triple Warmer 17

Inner side of the leg

Kidney 3

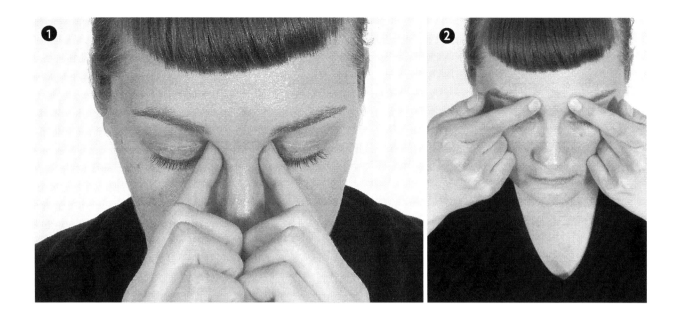

Eye Problems

Start your day with rolling your eyes. It is a good eye exercise: Sit on the chair and look straight forward. Then look – without turning your head – to the upper right corner of the room and then to the lower right corner. Next turn your eyes to the lower left corner of the room and then to the higher left corner. Look as far as you can without turning your head. Repeat the series many times. Change the direction and repeat the same. Then refresh your eyes by rubbing your palms together and placing them over the eyes.

Here is what to do to stimulate your eyesight with acupressure:

1. Start by pressing the point Bladder 1 in the inner corner of the eye. The pressure must be extremely gentle.

2. Place your fingers on the inner or medial extremity of the eyebrow. The point Bladder 2 is located on the upper corner of the eye socket. Press up toward the bone. It is easier to press if you tilt your head down and let it relax onto your forefingers.

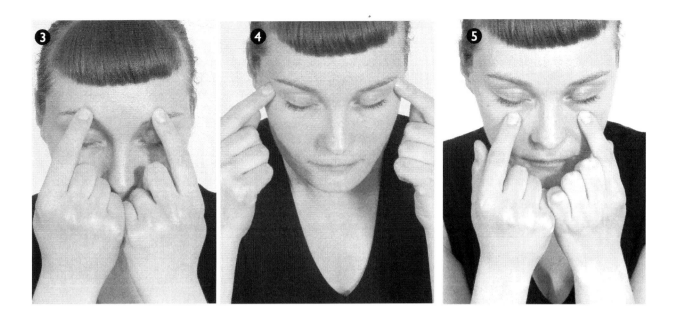

3. Place your fingers directly above the pupil, in the middle of the eyebrow. Here is located the point Yuyao. Press on the point.

4. Move your fingers from the eyebrow over the ridge of the temporal bone to the point Gallbladder 1. Press on the point gently.

5. Place your fingers in a very small hollow in the cheek bone, about one finger width downward from the eye socket, in a direct vertical line with the pupil. Here is the point Stomach 2. Press on the point gently.

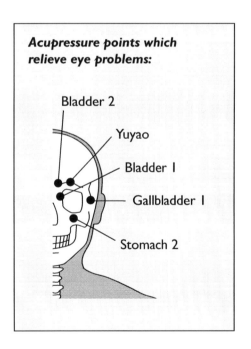

Acupressure points which relieve eye problems:

Bladder 2

Yuyao

Bladder I

Gallbladder I

Stomach 2

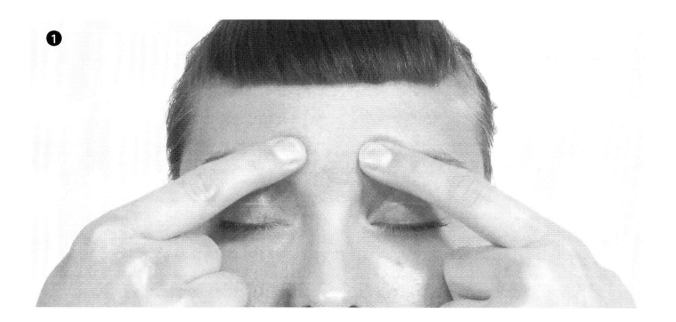

①

Flu

Traditional Chinese medicine calls flu "wind" or "evil wind." When the weather is cold, the Chinese doctor tells his patient "to close the gates of wind" by protecting his neck with a scarf.

Acupressure does not cure the flu, but it helps you get better more quickly by stimulating your own immune system. At first it may even seem that the flu is worsening, as the pressure on the points increases the mucus secretion while relieving nasal congestion.
Here is what to do:

1. Place your fingers on the inner or medial extremity of the eyebrow. The point Bladder 2 is located there, above the upper corner of the eye socket. Press up toward the bone. It is easier to press if you tilt your head down and let it relax onto your fore fingers.

2. Place your fingers beside your nostrils underneath the cheekbones. There you will find the point Large Intestine 20. Press up toward the bone. It relieves nasal congestion.

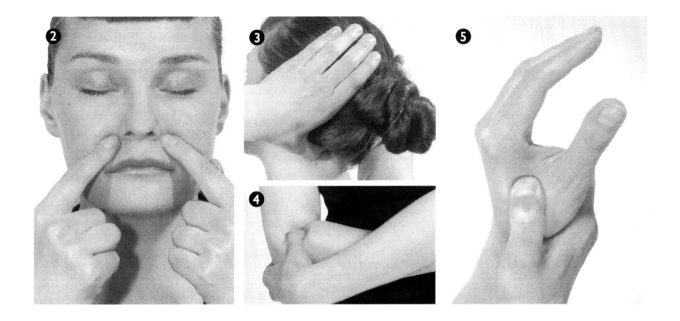

3. Place both of your thumbs underneath the base of your skull. The point Gallbladder 20 is located in the depression between the sternocleidomastoideus and trapezius muscles. Tilt your head back to relax it on your thumbs and press firmly up toward the bone. Keep the pressure steady, do not massage or rub. If you feel pain radiating to the forehead, keep pressing until the pain disappears.

4. Bend your elbow. Press with your thumb at the end of the elbow crease on the outside of your forearm. This is Large Intestine 11. It relieves fever and infection.

5. Press with your thumb in the web on the back of your hand, between the thumb and the forefinger. This point is Large Intestine 4, the best-known point for aches and flu in traditional Chinese medicine. Press toward the bone that connects with your index finger.

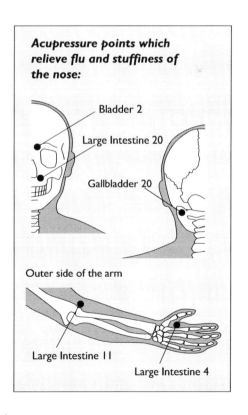

Acupressure points which relieve flu and stuffiness of the nose:

Bladder 2

Large Intestine 20

Gallbladder 20

Outer side of the arm

Large Intestine 11

Large Intestine 4

Frozen Shoulder

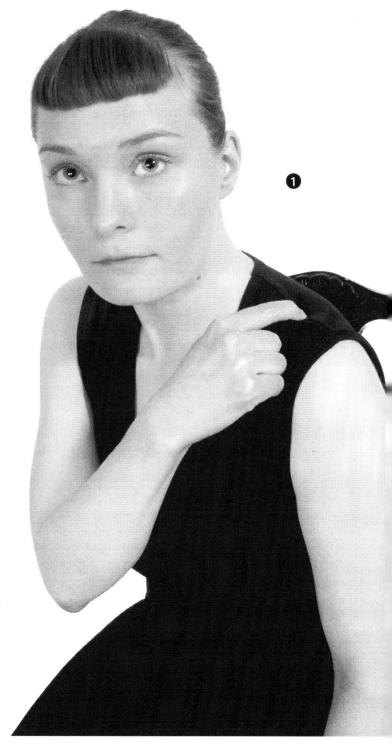

Frozen shoulder is usually caused by an external injury in younger people. In older people it is a sign of aging. It is an inflammation of the rotator cup and its peripheral area. It usually starts with a dull pain or aching in the shoulder joint, then proceeds to a very painful condition in which the range of motion of the arm is very limited.

Try to move the arm even if it feels painful. It makes the healing faster. Hold something heavy with your hand, a hand weight or a cast iron frying pan. Bend your body a little bit forward and swing your arm in several directions. Do this many times a day to keep the joint loose and flexible.

First release the shoulder tension by tapping both shoulders with a fist several times back and forth. Then:

1. Find with your forefinger a tender point in the shoulder muscle in the middle between

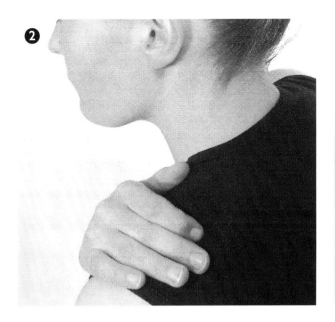

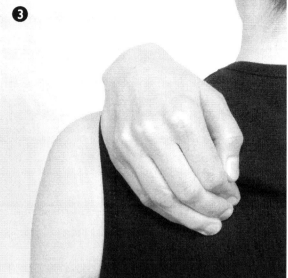

the base of the neck and the end of the shoulder. This point is Gallbladder 21. When you dig with your finger deep in the muscle, you'll find there a depression. The point is in this depression. Press on the point and hold the pressure until the pain subsides. Remember: do not press behind the shoulder muscle but right at the top of it.

2. Move your finger from Gallbladder 21 backward, behind the shoulder muscle. The point Triple Warmer 15 is located in the depression above the shoulder blade. Press on the point.

3. Place your palm on the shoulder blade. Almost in the middle of the shoulder blade is a tender area. This is Small Intestine 11. Press on the point with your palm or fingers.

4. Place your finger just below the bulging muscle of the upper arm. It is about one third of the way from the shoulder down the arm. This point is Large Intestine 14. Feel with your finger until you find a tender spot and press on it.

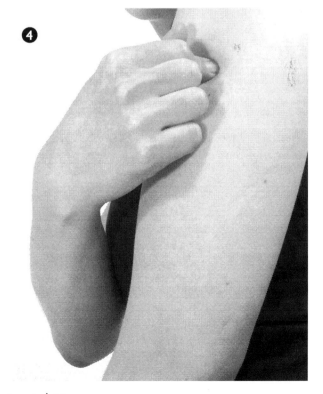

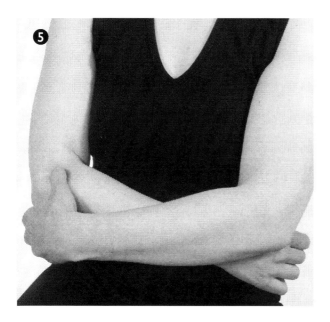

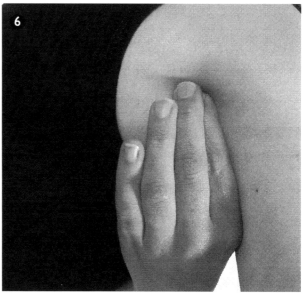

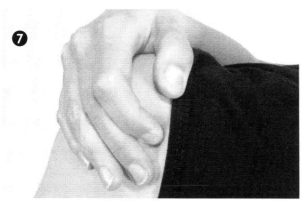

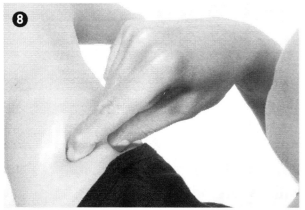

5. Bend your elbow. Press with your thumb at the end of the elbow crease on the outside of your forearm. This is Large Intestine 11. It relieves inflammation.

6. Lift your arm. Grab the muscle behind the armpit with your thumb and forefinger and press the fingers together. You are now pressing the point Small Intestine 9, which is located on the backside of the muscle.

7. Grasp your shoulder with your hand and press with your fore or middle finger on the acupressure point Small Intestine 10, which is located in the depression behind and below the point of the shoulder bone (the acromion process).

8. Stretch your arm slowly in a horizontal position and support it on the back of a chair. You'll now find two small depressions (Large Intestine 15 and Triple Warmer 14) between the tip of the shoulder and the triceps muscle. They are located at one inch from each other. Press on the points firmly with your thumb and forefinger

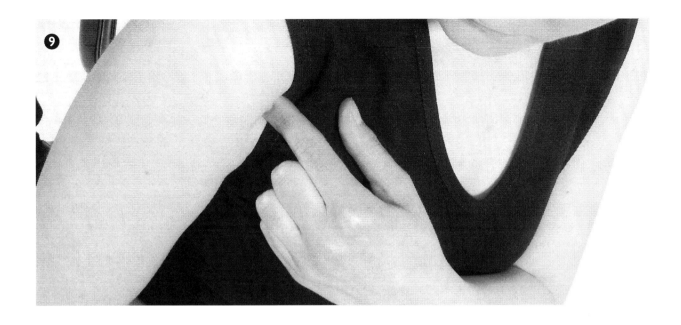

9. Feel with your finger between the upper arm and the pectoral muscle until you find a tender spot. Jianqian is located in the midpoint halfway between the armpit and the tip of the shoulder. Press on the point.

Finish the treatment by massaging the shoulder and pressing all the tender points.

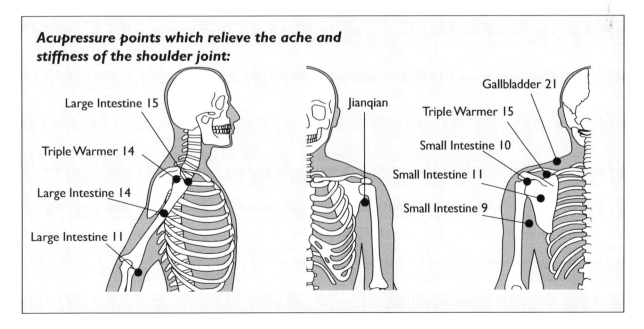

Acupressure points which relieve the ache and stiffness of the shoulder joint:

Large Intestine 15

Triple Warmer 14

Large Intestine 14

Large Intestine 11

Jianqian

Gallbladder 21

Triple Warmer 15

Small Intestine 10

Small Intestine 11

Small Intestine 9

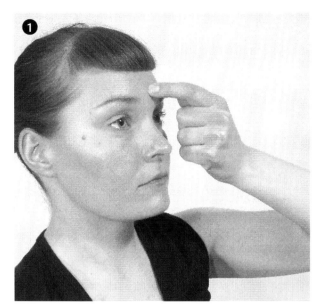 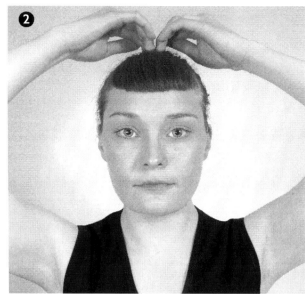

Headache

The most common cause of headache is tension in the neck and shoulders. When the hard, tense, and swollen muscles are pressing the blood vessels in the neck and shoulders, the supply of oxygen to the brain diminishes and the head starts to ache. Headaches can also be caused by flu, sinus problems, eye strain, hunger, stress, or even change in the weather.

A headache caused by the neck tension usually eases as soon as the muscles of the neck are relaxed by acupressure. You should, however, continue the treatment to prevent the recurrence of the aches.

Migraine headache is different. It starts when a stimulus triggers a reaction in which the blood vessels in the head enlarge. The ache is often one-sided and may last for days. Nausea and visual disorders are typical symptoms of the migraine headache. Migraine should be treated preventively, between the episodes, for acupressure might even worsen the condition if it is applied once the episode has already started.

You should consult a medical doctor if the headache is persistent or occurs daily.

If the headache is connected to the menstrual cycle, also press the points in the chapter Menstrual Irregularity and Cramps (p. 68).

Release the shoulder tension:

First release the shoulder tension following the instructions of the chapters Neck and Shoulder Tension and Pain (p. 74). You do not have to press all the points every time.

Rub the head:

1. Begin the treatment between the eyebrows on the forehead. Here is the point Yintang. It is an important calming point known by the yogis as the "third eye". Rub the point with circular movements.

2. Rub the forehead up toward the crown. In the middle of the crown is the point Du 20. You'll find the point by imagining two straight lines over the skull. One of the lines goes from one ear to another and the other from the nose to the back of the head. Du 20 is at the intersection of these lines. Rub Du 20 with your fingers. Then continue rubbing above and below the base of the skull.

Next, rub the hairline in front of the skull. Start from the middle and continue to the temples.

Release the muscles on the bottom of the skull:

When pressing the points in the neck, tilt your head back to rest on your thumbs and press firmly up toward the bone. Keep the pressure steady, do not massage or rub. If you feel pain radiating to the forehead, keep pressing until the pain disappears. Do not press directly on the bone.

3. Place both of your thumbs underneath the base of your skull in the middle of the tight muscles right next to the vertebra. The point Bladder 10 is located one thumb's width up from the posterior hairline. Press on the point.

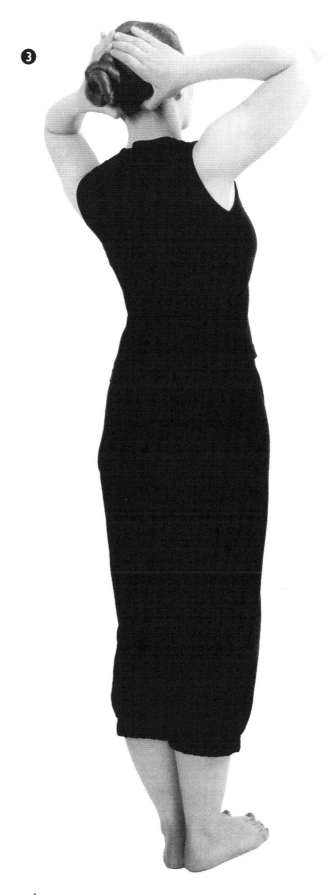

❸

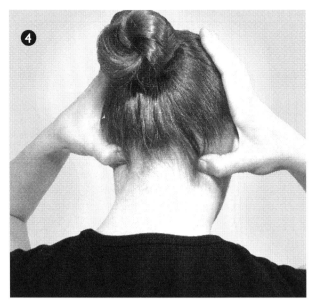

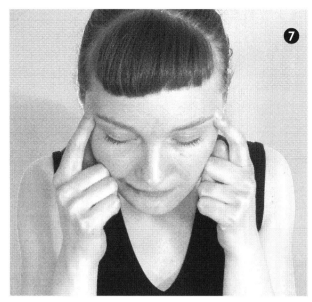

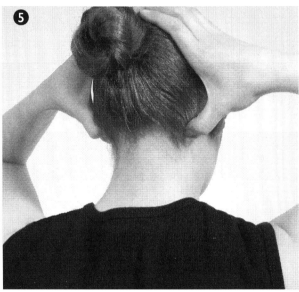

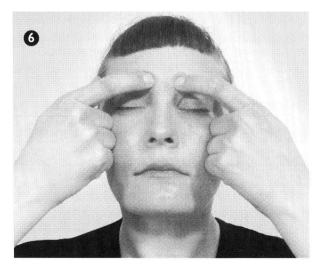

4. Move your thumbs outward along the base of the skull until you come to a depression. The point Gallbladder 20 is located in the depression between the sternocleidomastoideus and trapezius muscles. Press on the point.

5. Move your thumbs further outward along the base of the skull until you come to another depression, just before the end of the occipital bone. The point Gallbladder 12 is located here. Press on the point.

Press on the forehead and the temples:

6. Place your fingers on the inner or medial extremity of the eyebrows. The point Bladder 2 is located on the upper corner of the eye socket. Press up toward the bone. It is easier to press if you tilt your head down and let it relax onto your forefingers.

7. Use your forefingers to gently press on your temples on the point Taiyang.

8. At one thumb's width directly above the middle point of the eyebrows, in a direct vertical line with the pupil, you'll find a small depression in the frontal bone. Feel a tender spot on the bone. This is the point Gallbladder 14. Press on the point.

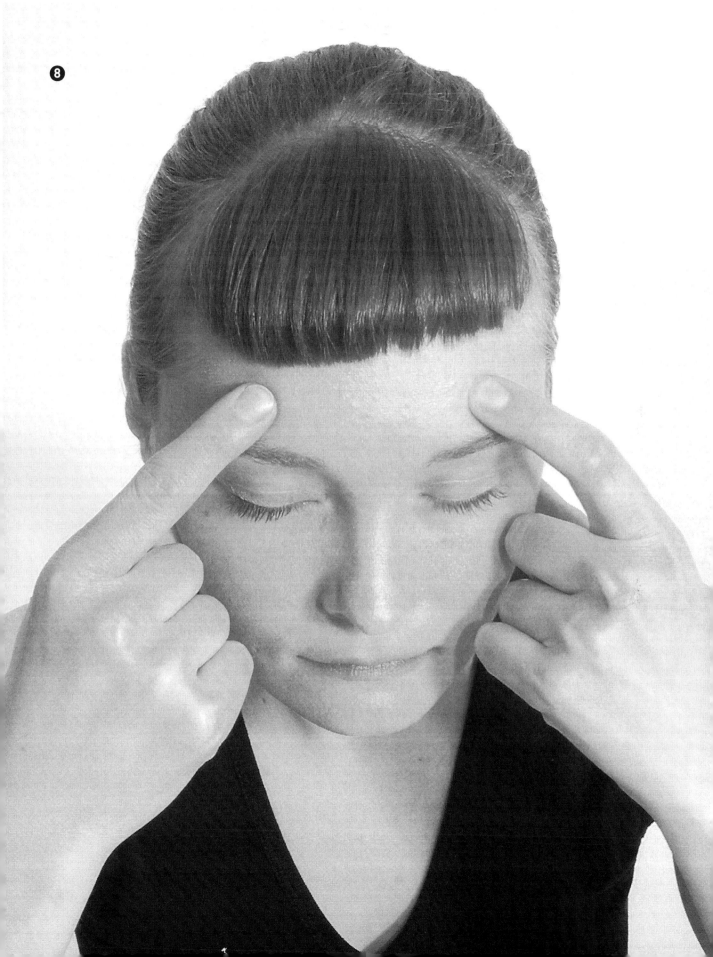

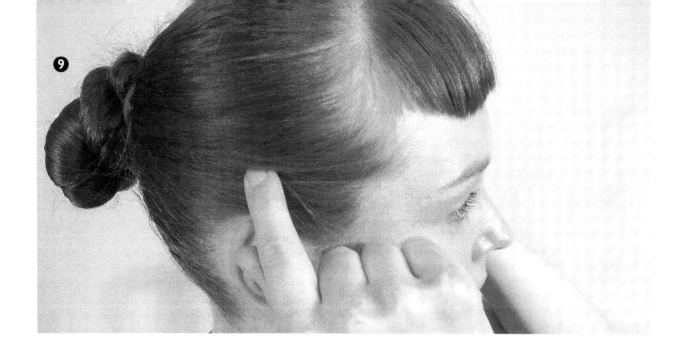

For migraine headache, also press the following points:

9. Rub your head around the ears with your finger-tips. Start at the frontal hairline and continue all the way to the bottom of the skull. You are rubbing many important points along the Gallbladder meridian. Repeat three times. Press on the point Gallbladder 8 at one thumb's width upward from the highest point of the ear. Use a very firm pressure against the skull.

If you do not wish to press acupressure points on the head, such as when you are in public, you may also treat headache using acupressure points located on other parts of the body:

10. Press with your thumb in the web on the back of your hand, between the thumb and the forefinger. This point is Large Intestine 4, the best-known point for all kinds of aches in traditional Chinese medicine. Press toward the bone that connects with your index finger.

11. If your headache is caused by stress: Sit on a chair and place your thumbs on top of the feet in the depression between the big and the second toe. This point is Liver 3, the basic point against irritability and stress. Hold a firm and steady pressure, even if the point feels very tender. Press simultaneously on both feet.

12. Press on the point Gallbladder 41 in the depression between the fourth and the little toe. Follow with your finger upward along the depression until you cross a tendon. Right next to the tendon you find a tender point. Press on that point.

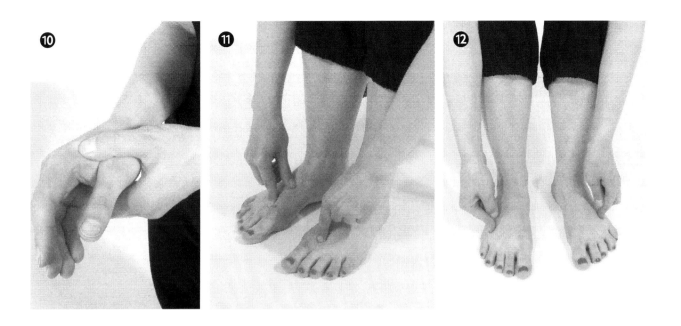

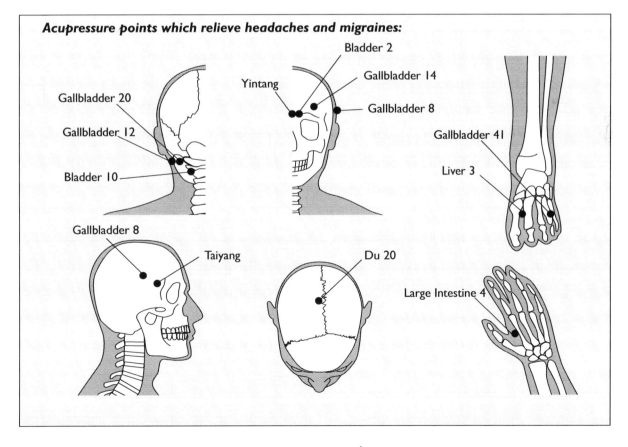

Acupressure points which relieve headaches and migraines:

Bladder 2

Gallbladder 14

Yintang

Gallbladder 8

Gallbladder 20

Gallbladder 12

Gallbladder 41

Bladder 10

Liver 3

Gallbladder 8

Taiyang

Du 20

Large Intestine 4

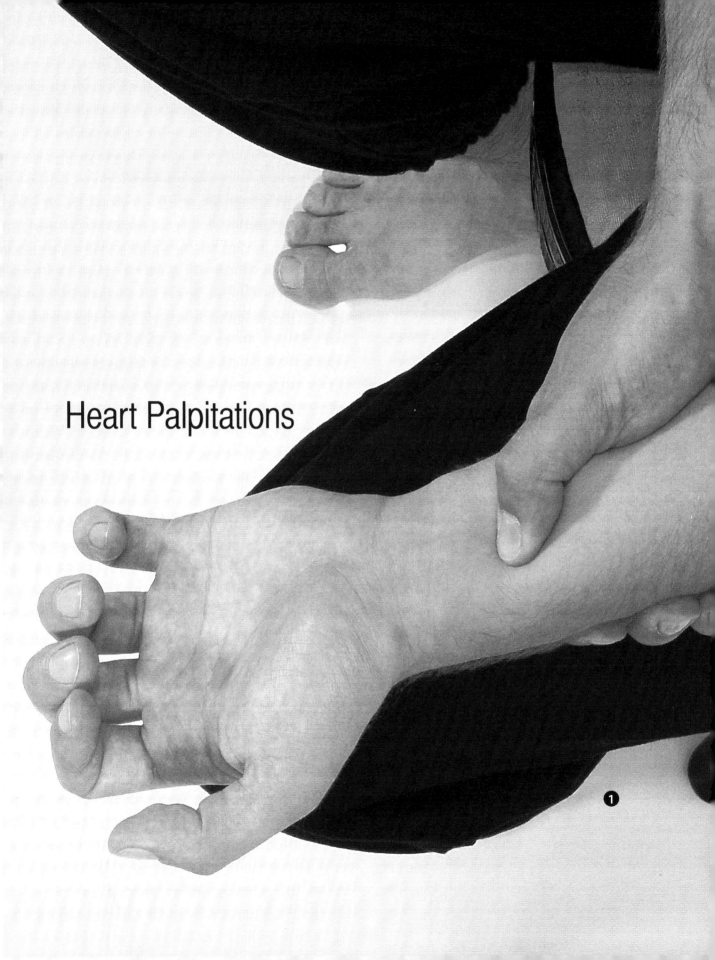

Heart Palpitations

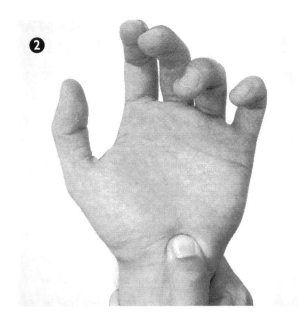

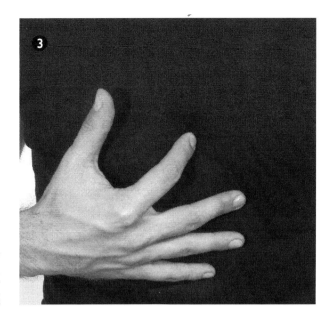

Acupressure can relieve the symptoms of heart disease even though it does not cure the illness itself. It calms the nerves and heart while improving the general health of the body. It is advantageous to use it to complement the usual medical treatment.

1. Press with the thumb of your right hand on the point Pericardium 6 on your left wrist. It is located in the middle of the inner side of the forearm, two thumbs' width from the wrist crease. Hold a firm pressure between the big tendons.

2. Press on the point Heart 7. You will find it by following along the palm with your finger the web between the ring finger and the little finger up to the wrist. The point is in the middle of the inside of the wrist crease, in the depression between the elbow bone and the carpal bone. Press on the point toward the carpal bone.

3. Place your finger in the middle of the front of the breastbone at the midpoint between the nipples. Find a tender area. This is the point Ren 17. Press on the point.

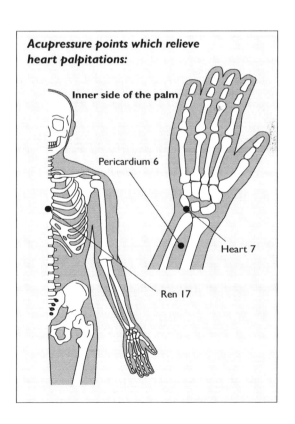

Acupressure points which relieve heart palpitations:

Inner side of the palm

Pericardium 6

Heart 7

Ren 17

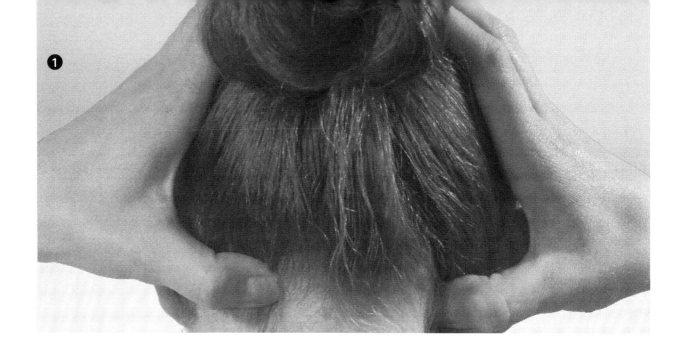

High Blood Pressure

In traditional Chinese medicine blood pressure problems are usually treated with herbal medicines. During treatment the patient is advised to practice daily relaxation and concentration exercises. The blood pressure is then gradually normalized, even if the treatment might last several months or even years. Both acupuncture and acupressure slightly lower blood pressure, but it rises again a few days after treatment. Sometimes Chinese doctors stroke carotid arteries in the neck in order to help decrease the blood pressure during the treatment. It must be done very carefully, one side of the neck at a time.

In the backside of the ear runs the "blood pressure line." According to traditional Chinese medicine, it lowers high blood pressure and raises low blood pressure. You can try this by rubbing the ears between your fingers.

There is no single point on the body that can bring about sudden reduction in blood pressure. The following points are for general balancing of the body, which gradually relieves the symptoms that occur as a result of high blood pressure.

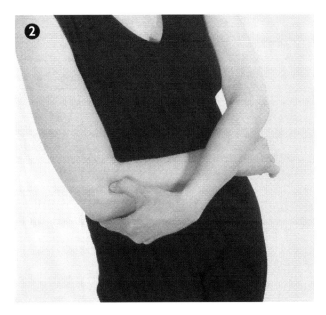

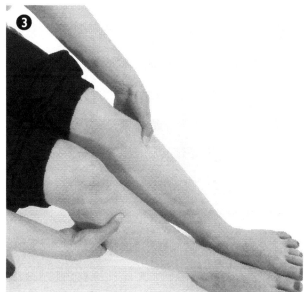

1. Place both of your thumbs underneath the base of your skull. Find the point Gallbladder 20, which is located in the depression between the sternocleido-mastoideus and trapezius muscles. Tilt your head back to relax on your thumbs and press firmly up toward the bone. Keep the pressure steady. Do not massage or rub.

2. Bend your elbow. Press with your thumb at the end of the elbow crease on the outside of your fore-arm. This is the point Large Intestine 11.

3. Sit on a chair and press on the point Stomach 36 which is located four fingers' width below the kneecap and one finger width on the outside of the shinbone.

4. Place your thumb on top of each foot in the de-pression between the big and the second toe. This point is Liver 3. Press on the point and hold a steady pressure for one minute.

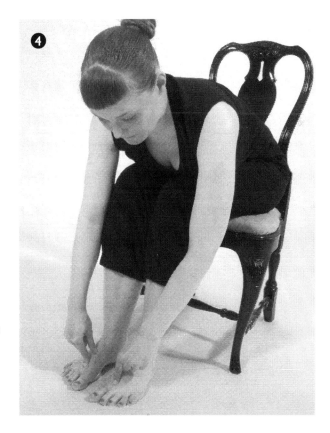

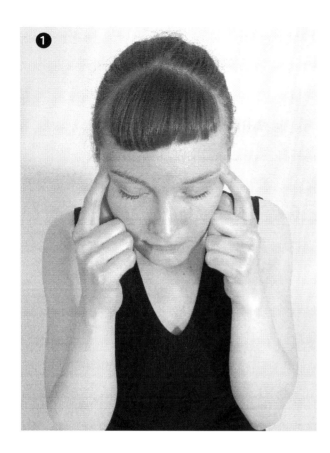

For symptoms caused by hypertension:

Headache:
1. Use your forefingers to gently press on your temples. Here is located the point Taiyang.

Ringing in the ears, insomnia and nervousness:
2. Press on the point Heart 7. You will find it by following with your finger the palm between the ring finger and the little finger up to the wrist. The point is in the middle of the inside of the wrist crease, in the depression between the elbow bone and the carpal bone. Press on the point toward the carpal bone.

3. Sit on a chair and press on the point Kidney 3. It is located midway between the inside of the ankle-bone and the Achilles tendon on the inner side of the ankle.

4. Press on the point Spleen 6. It is located on the inner side of the leg, at four fingers' width above the ankle and between the shinbone and Achilles tendon. Find a tender spot in the muscle very close to the bone, but not directly on it.

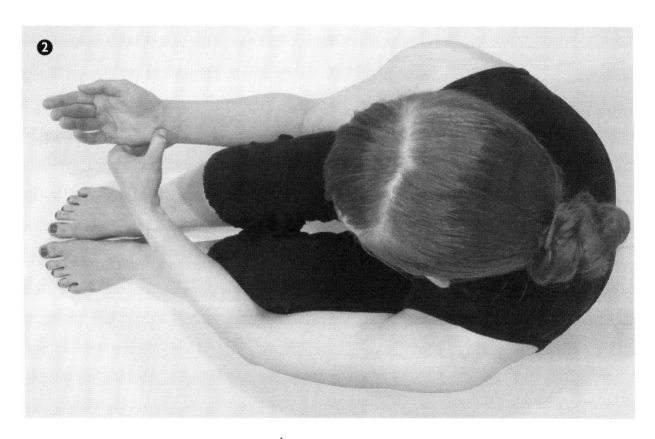

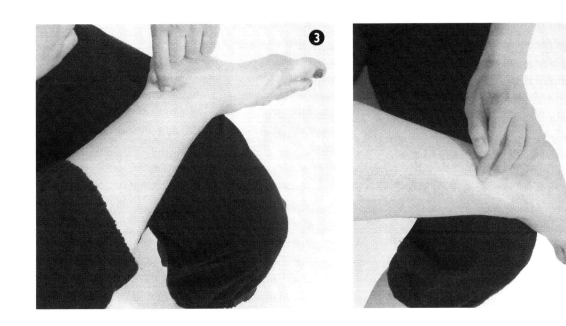

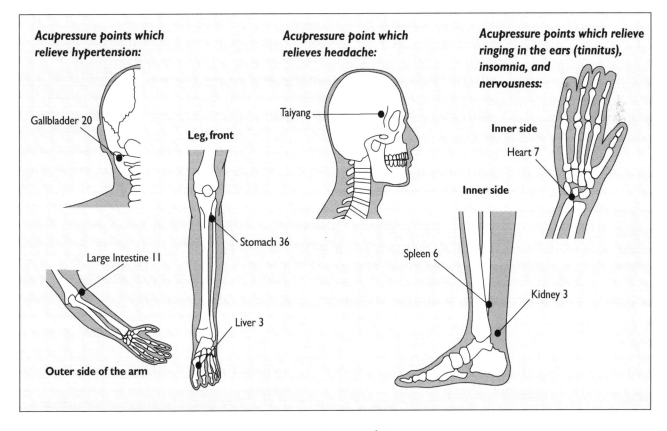

Acupressure points which relieve hypertension:

Gallbladder 20

Leg, front

Large Intestine 11

Stomach 36

Liver 3

Outer side of the arm

Acupressure point which relieves headache:

Taiyang

Acupressure points which relieve ringing in the ears (tinnitus), insomnia, and nervousness:

Inner side

Heart 7

Inner side

Spleen 6

Kidney 3

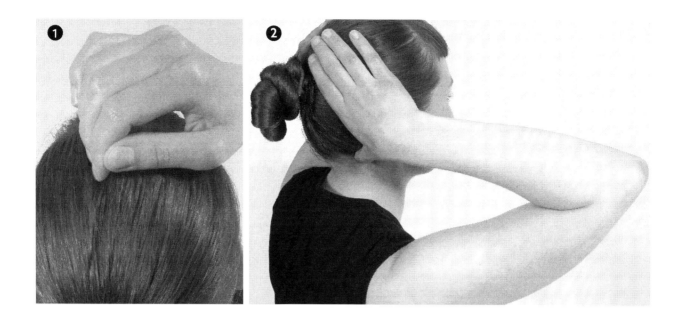

Hot Flashes and Menopausal Problems

Hot flashes and night sweats are common symptoms of menopause. About 70 percent of women experience them after the onset of menopause. The sweating disturbs the sleep at night causing irritability, memory and concentration difficulties the next day. In Traditional Chinese Medicine (TCM) these symptoms are called "Female hysteria". They can be reduced by avoiding coffee and alcohol, eating special foods like dates and walnuts, and preventing stress through exercise and meditation.

You can reduce the symptoms also by using the following acupressure points several times a day. You can also add some of the points from the chapter Menstrual Irregularity and Cramps (p. 40). You do not have to use all of the points every time.

1. Start by pressing the point Du 20 on the crown of the head. To find the point, imagine two straight lines over the head: one starting in the nape below the base of the skull and going over the crown to the middle of the eyebrows. The other leads from the

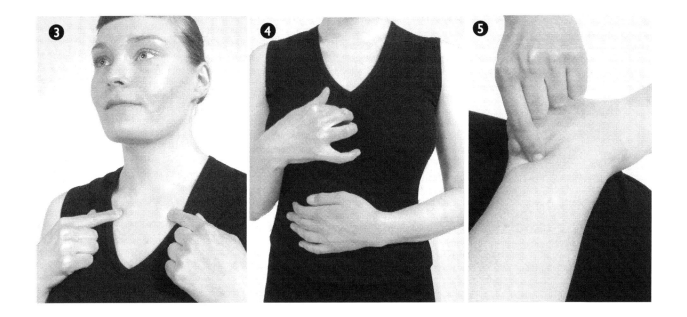

highest point of one ear to the highest point of the other. Du 20 is where these two lines cross.

2. Place both of your thumbs underneath the base of your skull. The point Gallbladder 20 is located in the depression between the sternocleidomastoideus and trapezius muscles. Tilt your head back to relax on your thumbs and press firmly up toward the bone. Keep the pressure steady, do not massage or rub. If you feel pain radiating to the forehead, keep pressing until the pain disappears.

3. Place your fingers in the hollows below the collarbone next to the breastbone. Press lightly on the point Kidney 27.

4. Find with your fingertips a tender point in the middle of the breastbone. It is located between the breasts at the level of the nipples. This is Ren 17, the Sea of Tranquility. Press on the point.

5. Press on the point Kidney 3 on the internal side of the ankle, in the hollow between the internal malleolus and the Achilles tendon.

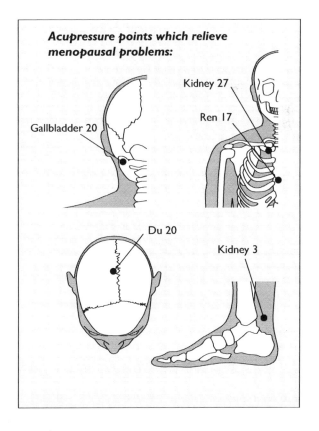

Acupressure points which relieve menopausal problems:

Kidney 27

Ren 17

Gallbladder 20

Du 20

Kidney 3

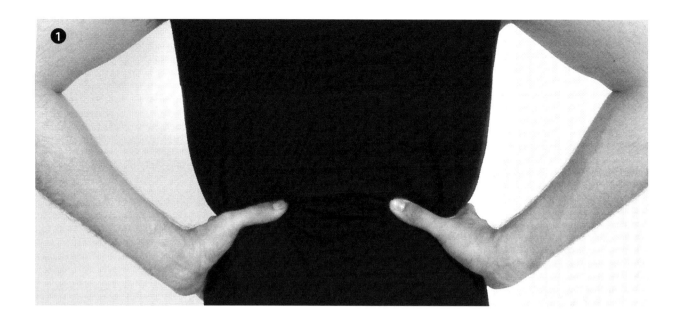

Impotence

Impotence is the most common sexual dysfunction in men of our times. Most men have experienced it in some period of their lives. Impotence can be caused by diabetes, obesity, hormonal imbalance, excess consumption of alcohol, addiction to stimulants or damage to the nerves. It can also be a side effect of blood pressure medications. Most common causes are, however, psychological: fatigue, stress or depression.

Good results have been achieved by acupuncture and acupressure in treating impotence for which an organic cause has not been found. Acupuncture can strengthen the body to improve sexual performance. The treatment should be done daily. Naturally a man must also try to improve his physical health and work on the issues that have caused or contributed to the problem.

1. Place both hands on the waist. On either side of the spine, one hand's width above the waist, in the middle of the long back muscle that is next to the spine, are located the points Bladder 23. They are important hormonal points, "the gates of life." Next, place your thumbs about one inch further out from

Acupressure points which treat impotence:

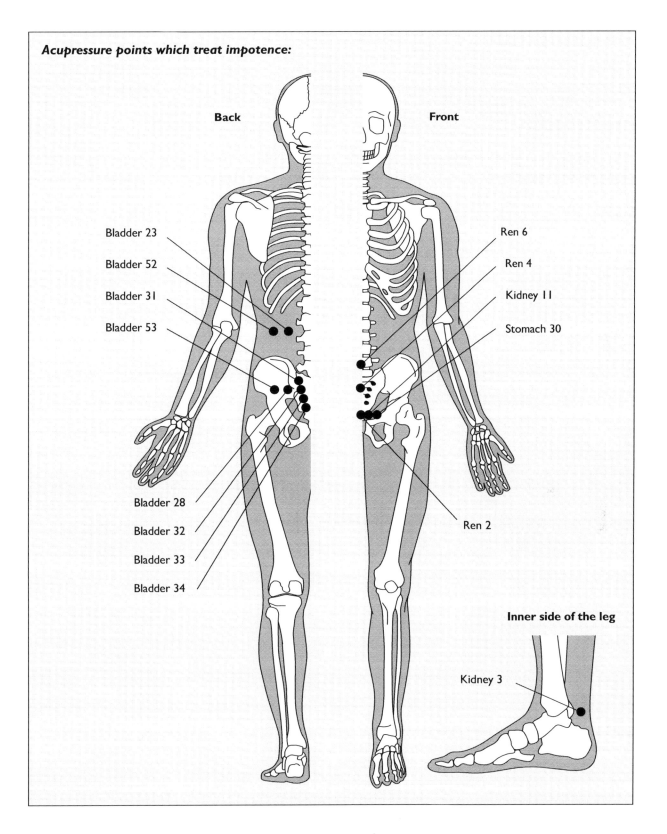

Back

Front

Bladder 23

Bladder 52

Bladder 31

Bladder 53

Bladder 28

Bladder 32

Bladder 33

Bladder 34

Ren 6

Ren 4

Kidney 11

Stomach 30

Ren 2

Inner side of the leg

Kidney 3

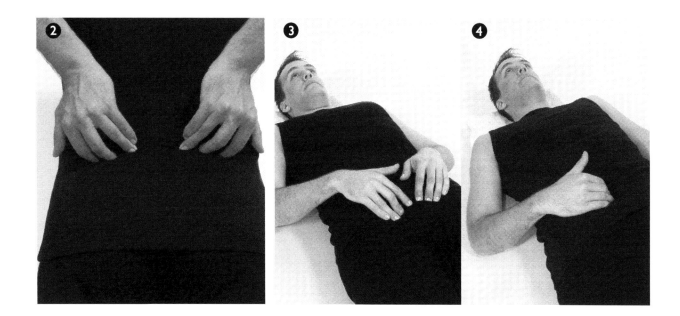

the spine in a horizontal line with Bladder 23. Here is located the point Bladder 52. Press on the points Bladder 23 and Bladder 52. You can also rub the whole area with your fists or curled hands. Next rub the sacrum with round, circular movements. You are stimulating the points Bladder 31, 32, 33, and 34, which are located in the middle on the sacral bone, in tiny depressions in the sacrum on both sides of the median line of the sacrum.

2. Firmly press on Bladder 32 in the second to the topmost depression in the sacrum. Then press on Bladder 28 and 53, which are further from the median line in a horizontal line with Bladder 32. You can also press all the points at the same time with your fingertips.

3. Lie down on your back and place your fingers just above the pubic bone. Press on the points Ren 2, Kidney 11, and Stomach 30. They strengthen the man's sexual organs.

4. Place your finger two fingers' width below the belly button. Here is located the point Ren 6. Place another finger four fingers' width below the belly button. Here is located Ren 4. Press on the points lightly, gradually increasing the pressure.

5. Finish the treatment by pressing on the point Kidney 3. It is located in the depression midway between the inside of the anklebone and the Achilles tendon on the inner side of the ankle.

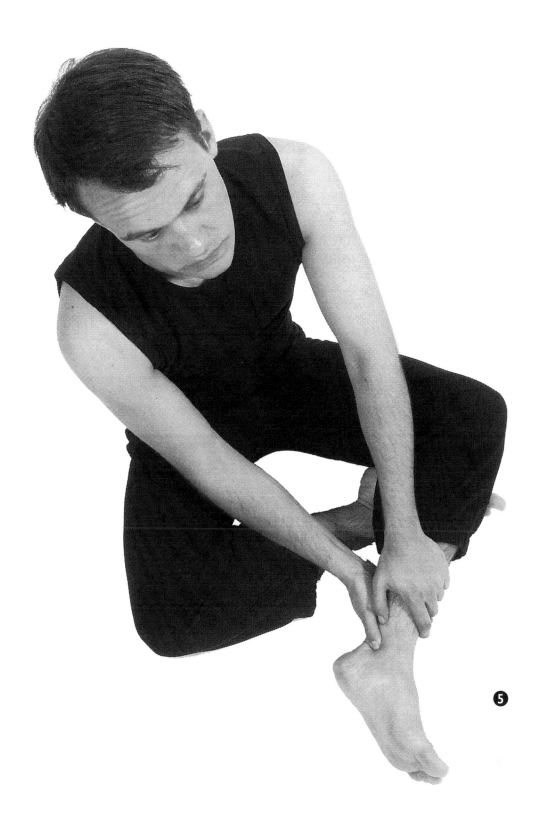

⑤

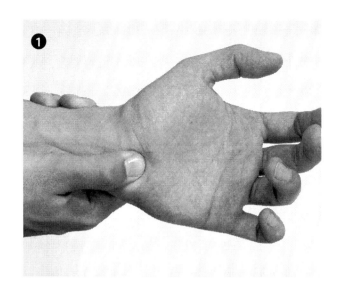

Insomnia

Very often people who complain of insomnia are afflicted with psychological problems, stress, worry, or anxiety that keep them awake at night. But there are also other reasons for insomnia. ate dinner, consumption of alcohol or coffee, hunger, pain, flu, and disturbances in digestion can temporarily prevent us from falling asleep.

Acupressure balances the body and mind and is an efficient way to treat insomnia. However, several months of acupressure is needed to change the sleeping pattern. If sleep does not come one night, it will do no good to start pressing the points right away. It is better to relax and start the treatments on the following day.

The following acupressure points are the basic points for insomnia. Press them daily. If the cause of the insomnia is anxiety or tension, use also the points from the chapter on Depression and Anxiety (p. 18).

1. Press on the point Heart 7. You will find it by following with your finger along the palm between the ring finger and the little finger up to the wrist. The point is in the middle of the inside of the wrist

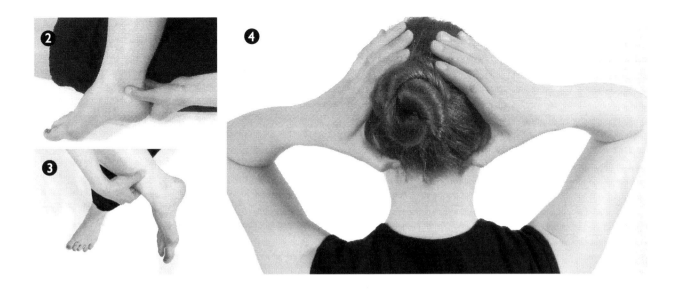

crease, in the depression between the elbow bone and the carpal bone. Press on the point toward the carpal bone.

2. Sit on a chair and press on the point Kidney 3 in the rear part of the inside of the ankle, in the hollow between the internal malleolus and the Achilles tendon.

3. Press on the point Spleen 6. It is located on the inner side of the leg, at four fingers' width above the ankle, between the shinbone and Achilles tendon. Find a tender spot in the muscle very close to the bone, but not directly on it.

4. Place both of your thumbs underneath the base of your skull. First find the point Gallbladder 20, which is located in the depression between the sternocleidomastoideus and trapezius muscles. Move your thumbs one finger width outward along the base of the skull, into a big muscle. This is the location of the point Anmian, "sleep well." It is the basic point for the insomnia. Tilt your head back to relax on your thumbs and press on Anmian firmly up toward the bone. Keep the pressure steady.

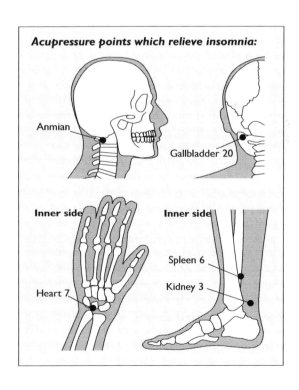

Acupressure points which relieve insomnia:

Anmian

Gallbladder 20

Inner side

Inner side

Spleen 6

Kidney 3

Heart 7

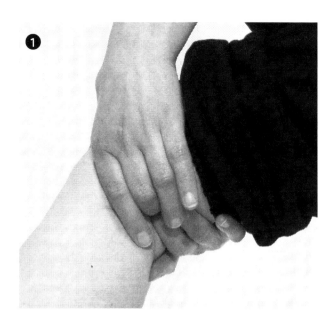

Knee Problems

The knee joint is the biggest joint in the body. As it is usually under a heavy strain, it is easily susceptible to wear, tear, and accidents. When the knee hurts, we instinctively hold it straight while walking. This tightens the back, thigh and calf muscles, the body gets gradually out of balance, and the pain starts to reflect to many other parts of the body. The pain in the back and foot muscles will usually also subside when the pain and swelling in the knee is relieved.

Press the following points many times a day for two or three weeks. Keep the knee warm during the treatment.

Sit on a chair and bend your knee. Start the treatment by relaxing the thigh and calf muscles by rubbing them vigorously. Then rub the knee with circular movements to improve the blood circulation and create friction.

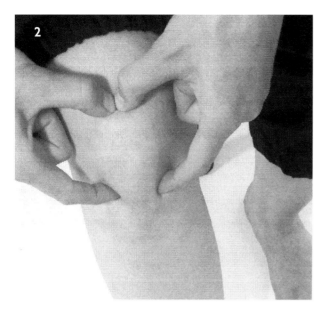

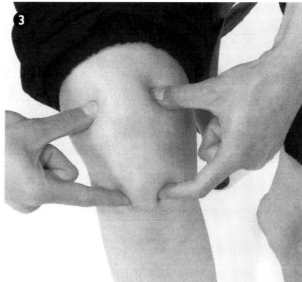

1. Press with the middle fingers of both hands in the center of the back of the knee in the middle of the crease of the knee joint. This is the point Bladder 40.

2. Press with the middle or forefingers on the soft cartilages directly under both sides of the kneecap, in the depression between the kneecap and the end of the shinbone. This is Stomach 35. Press upward toward the kneecap. Press at the same time with your thumbs on the point Heding directly above the upper edge of the kneecap.

3. Hold the pressure with your forefingers on Stomach 35 on both sides below the kneecap and place the thumb of one hand obliquely upward to the outer side of the quadriceps (the front thigh muscle) on the point Stomach 34. Place the thumb of the other hand obliquely upward to the inner side of the thigh muscle on the point Spleen 10. Press on all of the four points at the same time.

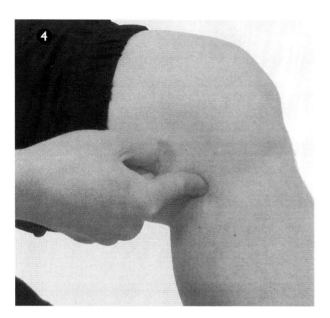

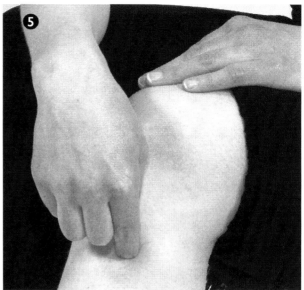

4. Feel the ligaments and muscles in the crease of the knee, on the inner side of the thigh. The point Liver 8 is located in the area where the crease ends, when the knee is bent. Press on the point and surrounding tender muscles.

5. On the outer side of your leg, right below the knee, you find heads of two bones, tibia and fibula. Gallbladder 34 is located at one thumb's width down from the midpoint between the heads of the bones. Press on the point.

6. Feel for a big knob below the kneecap, on the inner side of the leg. This is the head of the shinbone. Directly below the head you'll find a very tender area. This is the point Spleen 9. Press on the point.

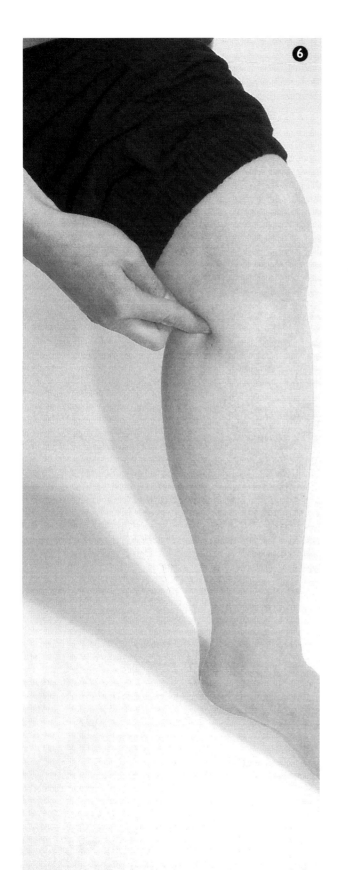

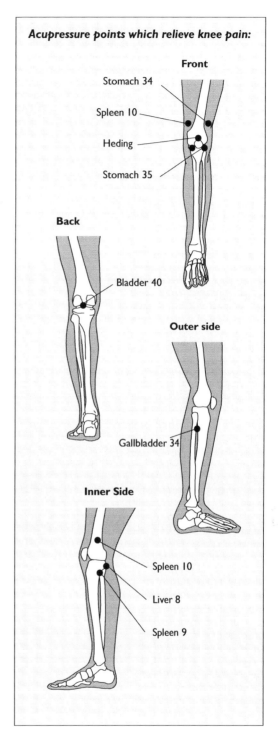

Acupressure points which relieve knee pain:

Front

Stomach 34

Spleen 10

Heding

Stomach 35

Back

Bladder 40

Outer side

Gallbladder 34

Inner Side

Spleen 10

Liver 8

Spleen 9

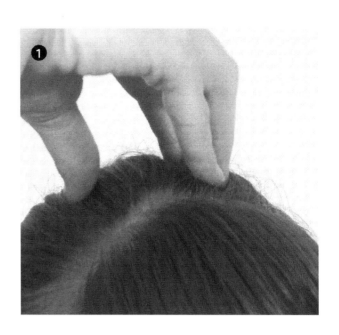

Memory and Concentration Difficulties

Memory and concentration gets worse under stress or when we have not got adequate sleep. It can also be caused by imbalance in blood sugar or lack of fluid in the body. The first thing to improve your thinking is to eat small meals frequently, drink enough water and sleep at least eight hours a night. The tension in the neck and shoulder muscles can also contribute to problems in memory. The tight muscles inhibit the blood circulation to the brain, which needs adequate supply of oxygen to function properly.

In addition to the points of this chapter, you should use the acupressure points illustrated in chapter Neck and Shoulder Tension and Pain (p 52).

1. Start by pressing the point Du 20 on the crown of the head. To find the point, imagine two straight lines over the head: one starting in the nape below the base of the skull and going over the crown to the middle of the eyebrows. The other leads from the highest point of one ear to the highest point of the other. Du 20 is where these two lines are crossing

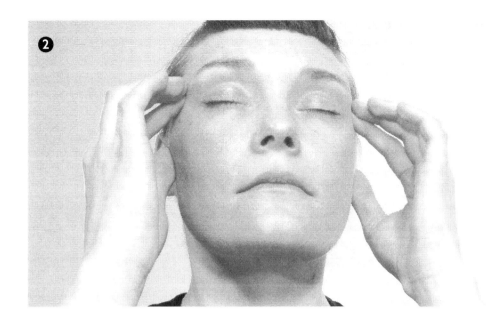

each other. One thumb width to front, back and both sides of this point you find a group of four points that is called Sishencong. These five points, Du 20 and Sishencong, improve memory and concentration. Press, rub or scratch the area.

2. Use your forefingers to gently press on your temples. Here is located the point Taiyang.

3. Place the tip of your right forefinger lightly between your eyebrows, where you find a strong energy point Yintang, called by yogis "the third eye." Place the tip of your left forefinger on the point Du 26 between your upper lip and your nose. Press firmly on both points.

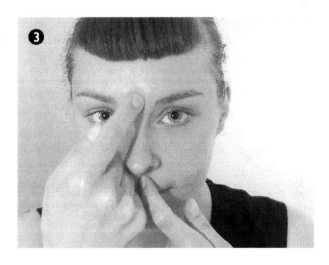

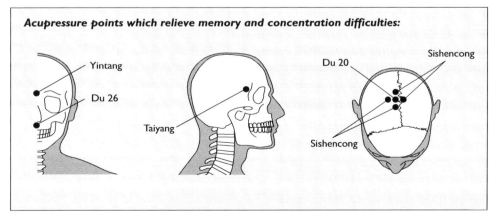

Acupressure points which relieve memory and concentration difficulties:

Yintang
Du 26
Taiyang
Du 20
Sishencong
Sishencong

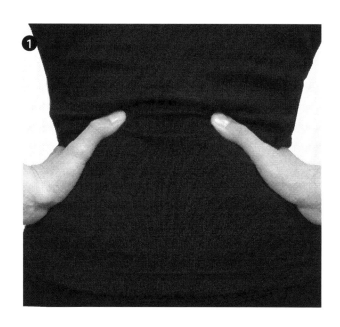

Menstrual Irregularity and Cramps

Menstrual problems can be a sign of an inflammation or hormonal imbalance. They can also be caused by stress, diet, emotions, and a change of the climate or life circumstances. Therefore it is important to eat healthy, get enough sleep and keep an even, balanced state of mind. During the menstruation it is good to place a heating pad or a warm compress on the stomach or the lower back when you are going to sleep. If the problems are serious or chronic, you should always consult a physician to determine the cause of the problem.

Daily acupressure stimulates and balances your hormones naturally. It takes a longer period to produce results than drugs, but has no side effects. Do not press on the points during menstruation.

1. Set both hands on your waist and press with your thumbs on the muscles along the spine. About one hand's width above the waist in your back, in the middle of the long muscle is the point Bladder 23,

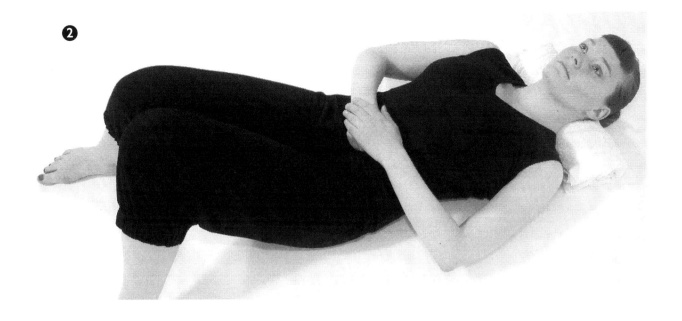

Sea of Vitality. It is an important hormonal point. Press on the point for 10 seconds.

2. Lie flat on your back and bend your knees. Place your fingertip in the center of your abdomen, about four fingers' width below the belly button. This is the point Ren 4. Place another finger about two fingers' width below the belly button on the point Ren 6. Press on both points and hold the pressure for a few minutes. Breathe deeply. You can also use the palm or loose fist if it feels more comfortable.

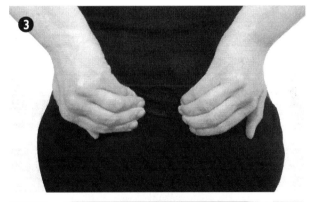

3. Find the points Bladder 31-34 in the sacrum. You'll find them in the following way: On both sides of the middle line of the sacrum you find a vertical line of four little holes in the bone. The points Bladder 31-34 are located in these holes. Rub or press the points with your fingertips. You can also rub the entire sacrum and press all the tender points on it.

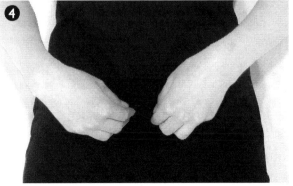

4. Place all your fingertips above your pubic bone. Press gradually inside and hold for a few minutes. Here are located the points Spleen 13, Stomach 29, Kidney 12 and Ren 3.

5. Sit on a chair and locate Spleen 10, the Sea of Blood, in the following way: Grab your left knee with your left hand so that the thumb is pointing to the soft muscle above the kneecap. You have found the point when you feel a very tender spot in the muscle. Press on the point.

6. Press on the point Spleen 6. It is located on the inner side of the leg, at four fingers' width above the ankle, between the shinbone and Achilles tendon. Find a tender spot in the muscle very close to the bone, but not directly on it.

7. If you get easily irritable before or during the menses, press on the point Liver 3. Place your thumbs on top of the feet in the depression between the big toe and the second toe. This point is Liver 3. Hold a firm and steady pressure, even if the point feels very tender.

❺

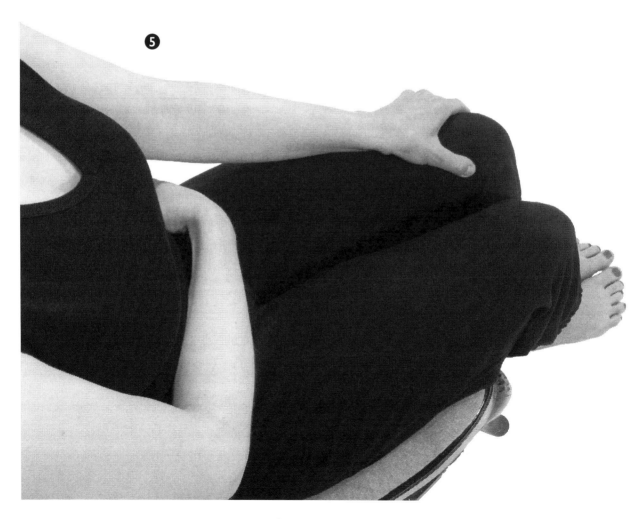

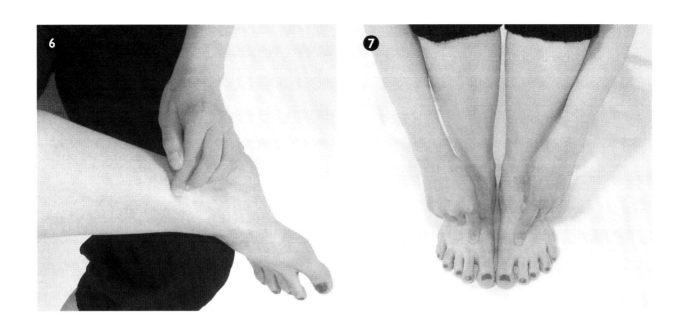

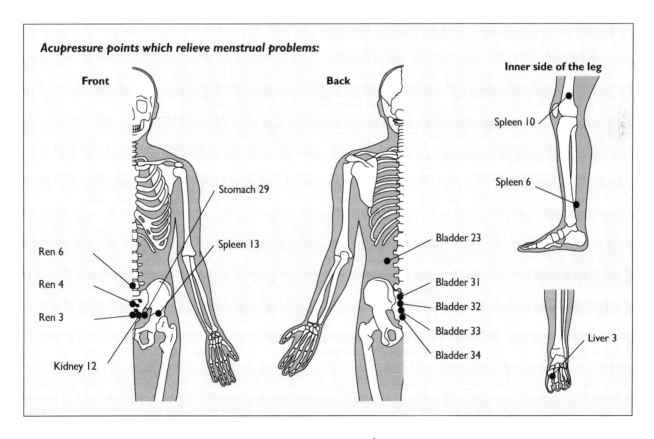

Acupressure points which relieve menstrual problems:

Front

Stomach 29

Spleen 13

Ren 6

Ren 4

Ren 3

Kidney 12

Back

Bladder 23

Bladder 31

Bladder 32

Bladder 33

Bladder 34

Inner side of the leg

Spleen 10

Spleen 6

Liver 3

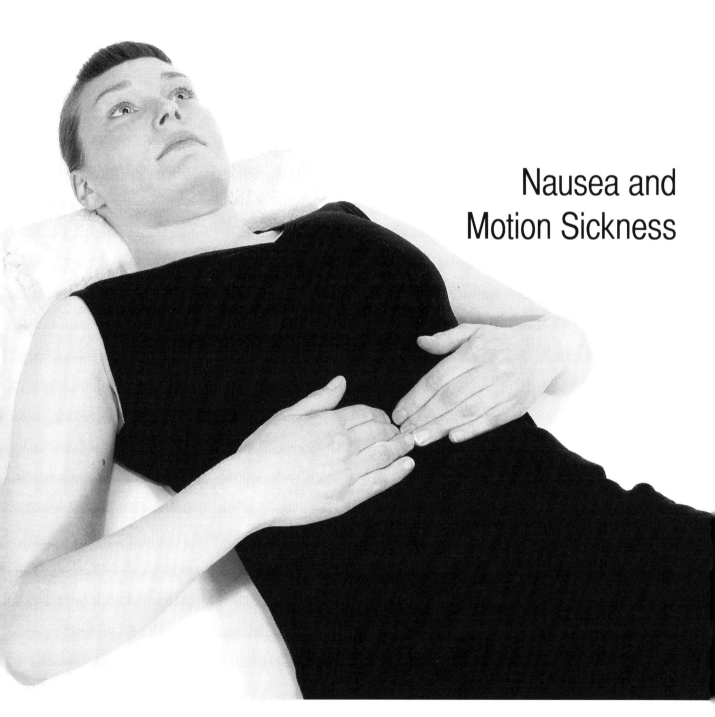

Nausea and Motion Sickness

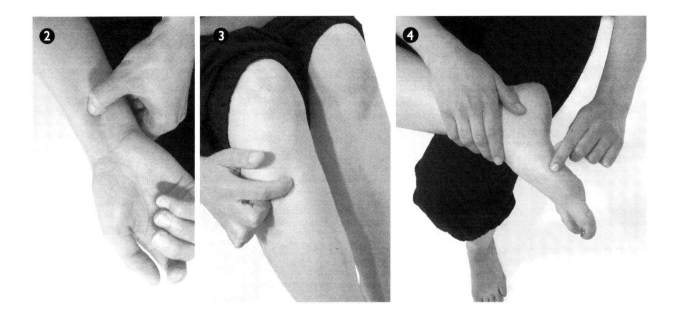

A simple way to treat nausea is to put a slice of raw ginger in the mouth and suck it until you feel better. If your child feels motion sickness you can press on the point between his or her eyebrows. This is the point Yintang, the well known calming point in traditional Chinese medicine, which the yogis call the "third eye". Usually, however, the ailment is treated by calming the stomach area.

1. Lie on your back with your knees bent. Place your fingertips at the midway between the lower end of your breastbone and your belly button. This is Ren 12, the calming point of the stomach. Press on the point with your fingertips and breathe deeply.

2. Press with your thumb on the point Pericardium 6 on the wrist. It is located in the middle of the inner side of the forearm, two thumbs' width from the wrist crease. Hold a firm pressure between the big tendons. This point calms the mind.

3. Sit on a chair. Place your finger on the point Stomach 36. It is located at four fingers' width below the kneecap, one finger width to the outer side of the shinbone.

4. Place your thumb in the arch of your foot, one thumb width from the ball of the foot toward the heel. Press on the point Spleen 4.

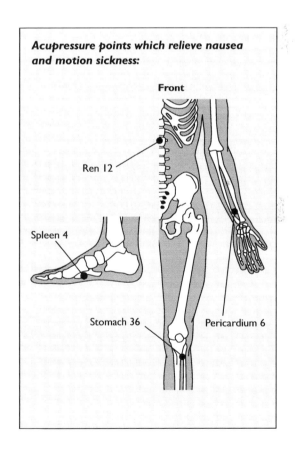

Acupressure points which relieve nausea and motion sickness:

Front

Ren 12

Spleen 4

Stomach 36

Pericardium 6

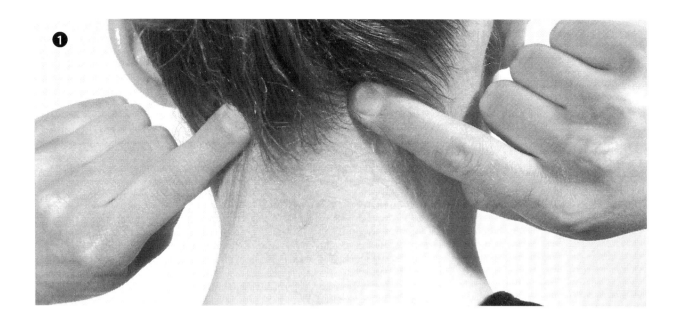

Neck and Shoulder Tension and Pain

Prolonged tension or overwork, stress, emotional problems, and lack of exercise or sleep might all be reflected as tensions and pains in the neck and shoulder area. This is the most common complaint of people who work with computers. If this is your case, you should press the following points daily to prevent the problem.

The following acupressure routine contains a lot of points, but you do not have to use all of them every time. Concentrate on the problem areas and press the points which feel most tender. Ask someone to help you if you cannot reach the points by yourself.

Neck and shoulders:
1. Place both of your thumbs underneath the base of your skull. The point Gallbladder 20 is located in the depression between the sternocleidomastoideus and trapezius muscles. Tilt your head back to relax on your thumbs and press firmly up toward the bone. Keep the pressure steady, do not massage or rub. If you feel pain radiating to the forehead, keep pressing until the pain disappears. Then rub your

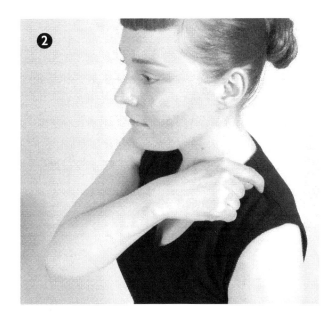

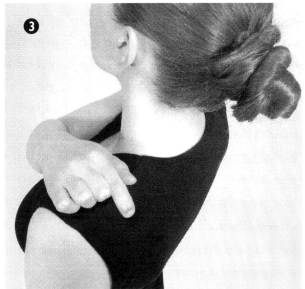

neck muscles with your fingertips and hit both of your shoulders lightly with clinched fists to relax your tight shoulder muscles.

2. Press with your forefinger on the sore point Gallbladder 21 in the trapezius shoulder muscle. It is the middle point between the base of the neck and the end of the shoulder. Press on the point and hold the pressure until the pain subsides. Do not press behind the shoulder muscle but right at the top of it.

3. Move your finger from Gallbladder 21 directly behind the shoulder muscle to the point Triple Warmer 15, which is located in the hollow directly above the shoulder blade. Press on the point. You can also press on the whole area with all your fingertips. There are several acupressure points above the shoulder blade. Keep the pressure steady, do not massage or rub.

4. Place your finger just below the bulging deltoid muscle of the upper arm. It is about one third of the way from the shoulder down the arm. This point is Large Intestine 14. Feel with your finger until you find a tender spot and press on it.

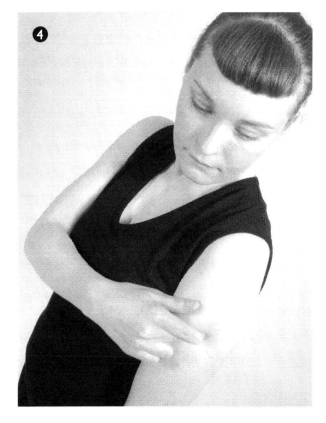

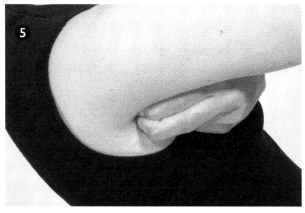

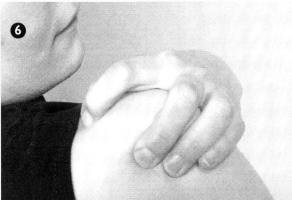

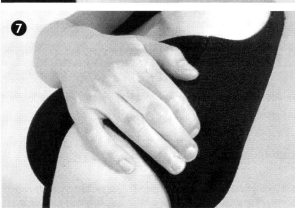

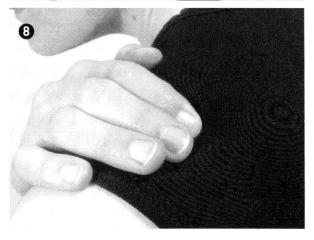

Upper back and shoulder blades:

5. Raise your arm. Grab with your thumb and your forefinger the muscle behind the armpit and press it. Feel the pain? You are now pressing on the point Small Intestine 9, which is located behind the muscle.

6. Grab your shoulder with your hand and place your middle finger behind the top of the shoulder in the depression below the external tip of the acromion process of the shoulder bone, on the point Small Intestine 10. Place your forefinger in a narrow depression above the bone on the point Large Intestine 16. Press on both points firmly.

7. Place your hand on your back. Almost in the middle of the shoulder blade is an area which is tender to touch. That is the point Small Intestine 11. Press on the point lightly with your fingertips.

8. Slide your finger straight upward, in the depression above the shoulder blade. This is the location of Small Intestine 12. Press on the point.

9. Place your finger in the upper corner of the shoulder blade, next to the spine. Find a tender, slightly swollen area. This is the location of Small Intestine 13. Press on the point.

10. Move your finger about one inch up and toward the spine. You'll feel a tight, small muscle (the levator scapulae), which lifts the shoulder blade. Two points, Small Intestine 14 and Small Intestine 15, are located on this muscle. Press on the points by pressing on the muscle with the forefinger and the middle finger as shown in the picture.

If the pain radiates along the arms:

After releasing the tension in the neck and shoulders, rub your arms and press on the following points:

11. Place your thumb on the point Triple Warmer 5. It is located in the middle of the outer side of the forearm, two thumbs' width from the wrist joint. Hold a firm pressure between the large bones. As there are several acupressure points located between the big bones, it is beneficial to press on the whole area.

12. Press with your thumb in the web on the back of your hand, between the thumb and the forefinger. This point is Large Intestine 4, the best-known point for aches and pain in traditional Chinese medicine. Press toward the bone that connects with your forefinger.

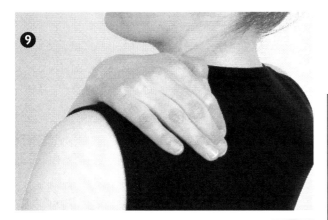

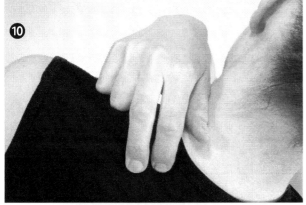

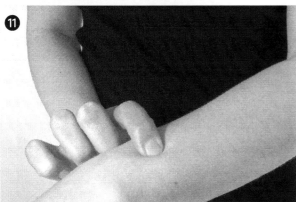

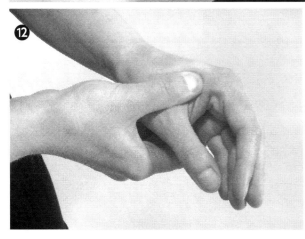

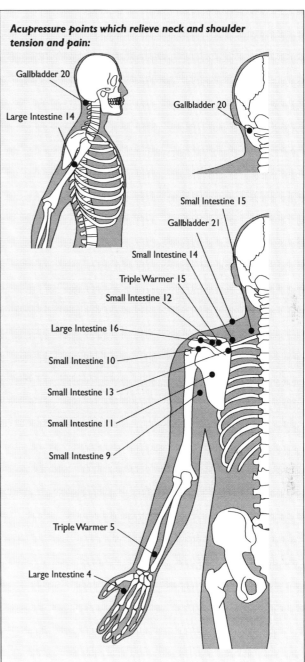

Acupressure points which relieve neck and shoulder tension and pain:

Gallbladder 20

Large Intestine 14

Gallbladder 20

Small Intestine 15

Gallbladder 21

Small Intestine 14

Triple Warmer 15

Small Intestine 12

Large Intestine 16

Small Intestine 10

Small Intestine 13

Small Intestine 11

Small Intestine 9

Triple Warmer 5

Large Intestine 4

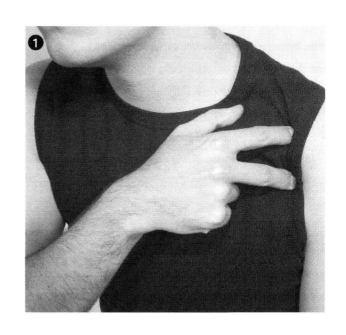

Numbness and Pain in the Arms

Aching and numbness of the arms is often caused by poor peripheral circulation of blood. Muscles are aching because they are not getting enough oxygen. The nerves leading from the neck to the arms might also be pinched or pressed by worn vertebrae in the neck or muscles too tight in the shoulder. The cause of the problem can also be one-sided work posture or static movement while working on the computer. The wrist bones press the nerves, the wrist gets inflamed and the pain spreads gradually to the whole arm.

While treating the numbness and pain one must thus first find out its origin. It is also beneficial to press the acupressure points indicated in the chapters Neck and Shoulder Tension and Pain (p. 52) or Wrist Pain (p. 70). You do not have to press all the points every time.

Press the following points several times a day Start by massaging both arms from tips of the fingers to shoulders. Remember to rub each of the fingers separately.

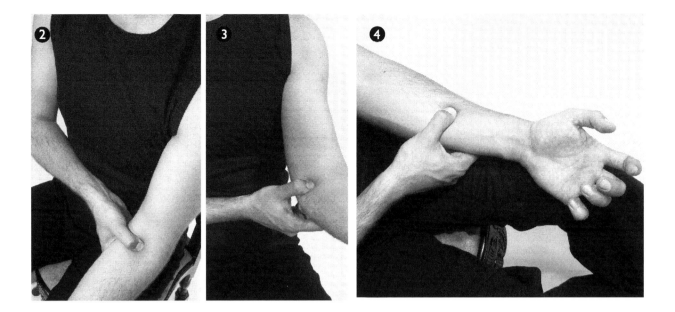

1. Slide your forefingers along the muscle below the collarbone toward the shoulders. Point Lung 2 is located in a small depression in the outer portion of the chest muscle just before the shoulder joint. Find the sensitive point below the end of the collarbone. Three fingers' width directly below Lung 2 is another tender point, Lung 1. You may find both points by pressing the outer portion of the chest muscle firmly with your fingers until you find sensitive points below your collarbone. Press both points simultaneously with your middle and forefingers.

2. Bend your elbow. In the groove of the elbow, on the outer side of the big tendon you'll find the point Lung 5. Press on the point with firm pressure.

3. In the groove of the elbow, on the inner side of the arm is an area which is very sensitive when touched. You'll find it by pressing the muscle. This is point Heart 3. Press on the point.

4. Press with the thumb of your right hand on point Pericardium 4 on your left forearm. It is located in the middle of the inner side of the forearm, halfway between the elbow and the wrist crease. Hold a firm pressure between the big tendons.

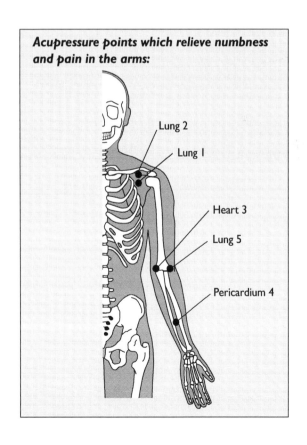

Acupressure points which relieve numbness and pain in the arms:

Lung 2

Lung 1

Heart 3

Lung 5

Pericardium 4

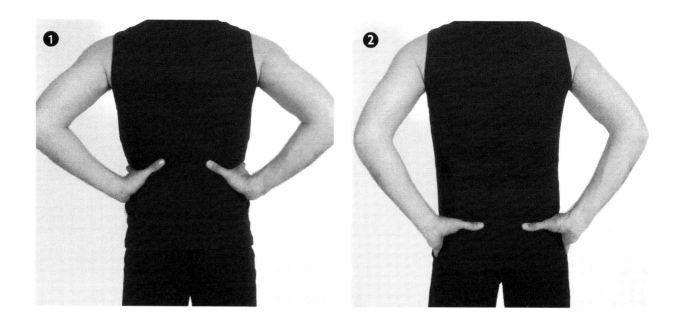

Prostrate Problems

The following points are used to treat inflammation of the prostate gland by acupuncture. You
can use the same points when treating yourself
with acupressure. Be prepared to be patient and
persistent. It might take a long time before you
get the results.

1. Place both of your hands on the waist. On
both sides of the spine in your back, about
one palm's width above the waist, in the middle of the long muscles, are the points Bladder
23, the Sea of Vitality. Start the treatment by
pressing on these points with the thumbs.

2. Find the points Bladder 28 and Bladder
32 in the sacrum. You will find them in
the following way: on both sides of the
vertical middle line of the sacrum you
will find four little holes in the bone.

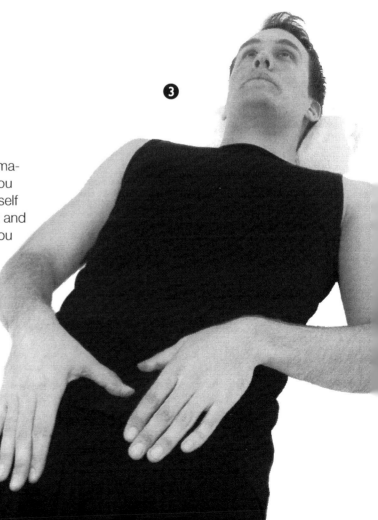

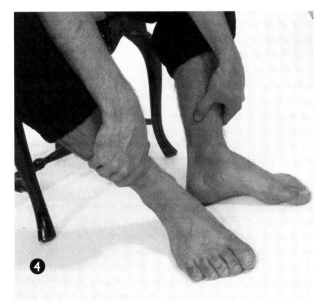

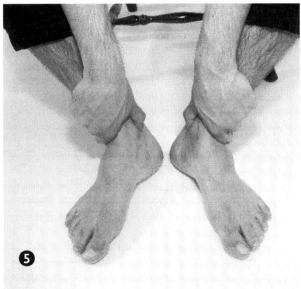

The point Bladder 32 is located in the second hole and Bladder 28 about one inch outward from Bladder 32. Rub or press on both points.

3. Put your finger in the middle of your belly, four fingers' width down from the navel. This is the point Ren 4. Put another finger one inch above the pubic bone. This is Ren 3. Press on both the points and hold for a few minutes. Breathe deeply.

4. Press on the point Spleen 6. It is located on the inner side of the leg, at four fingers' width above the ankle, between the shin- bone and Achilles tendon. Find a tender spot in the muscle very close to the bone, but not directly on it.

5. Press on the point Kidney 3 in the rear part of the inside of the ankle, in the hollow between the internal malleolus and the Achilles tendon.

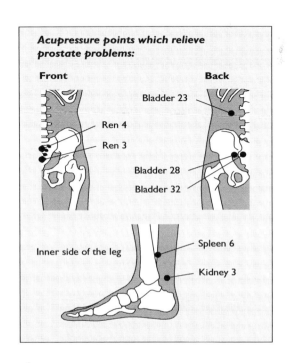

Acupressure points which relieve prostate problems:

Front   Back

Bladder 23

Ren 4

Ren 3

Bladder 28

Bladder 32

Inner side of the leg

Spleen 6

Kidney 3

Sciatica and Lower Back Pain

The sciatic nerve is the longest nerve in the body. It is formed from several lumbar and sacral spinal nerves. It passes at the back of the pelvis near the sacrum to the buttock, from where it runs down behind the back of the thigh to the lower leg and the foot. When the nerve is inflamed or pressed, one feels a sharp pain that sometimes extends from the buttock to the foot. The most common causes of sciatica are a herniated disk, aging, sitting a long time in the same position, cold and dampness.

For pains which are only temporary, acupressure is an efficient way to get relief. But if the pain is chronic, severe, and persistent, it needs an intensive physical examination because many illnesses have the same symptoms as sciatica.

Press the following points daily for several weeks. It is important that you keep the waist and the sacral areas warm during the time of the treatment.

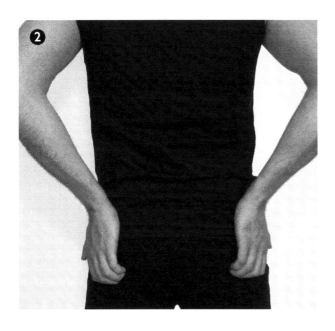

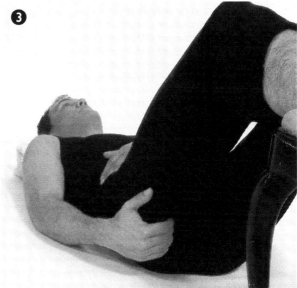

Follow these steps if you treat yourself.

First rub your lower back and sacral area with both hands.

1. Place both of your hands on the waist. On both sides of the spine, about one palm's width above the waist, in the middle of the long muscle of the back or latissimus dorsi, you find the point Bladder 23. Start the treatment by pressing with your thumbs on this point. Do not press too hard. Continue downward, pressing the muscle, an inch at a time, until you come to the middle of the sacrum (points Bladder 23-27). Repeat three times.

2. Grasp your buttocks and press on the point Gall-bladder 30 with your knuckles. It is in the big gluteus muscle on the cheek of the buttock. Press hard, until you find a tender area. You can also press the point by lying on your back and placing the wrists underneath your buttocks.

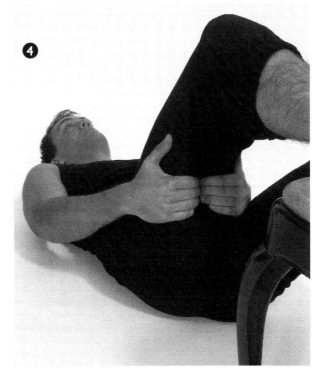

3. Lie on your back and raise your legs on a chair. Grab your legs with your fingers just below your buttocks, in the middle of the big muscle behind the thigh. This is the point Bladder 36. Pull the muscle toward the buttocks.

4. Continue lying on your back with your legs bent and press the point Bladder 37. You'll find it in the middle of the rear part of the thigh, halfway between the buttock and the knee.

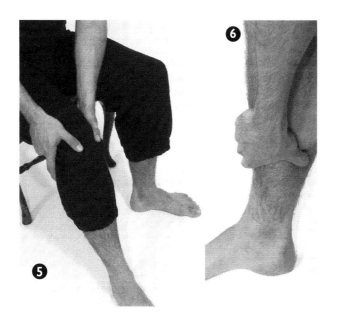

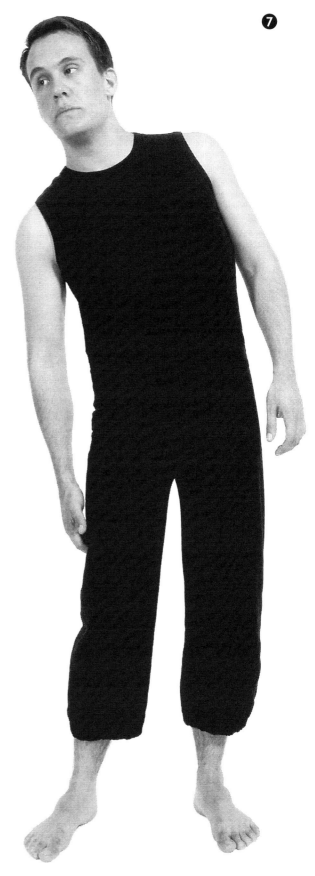

5. Sit on a chair and press on the point Bladder 40 in the center of the groove behind the knee. Do not press too hard.

6. Place your fingers at the point where the calf muscle bulge joins the Achilles tendon. Keep pressing around the area until you find a tender point. This is Bladder 57. Press on the point.

7. Stand up and let your arms hang to the side. The point Gallbladder 31 is located where the tip of your middle finger touches the thigh muscle, on the posterior border of the femur or thigh bone. Find a tender area and press there.

8. Sit on a chair. On the outer side of your leg, right below the knee, you find the heads of two bones, tibia and fibula. Gallbladder 34 is located at one thumb's width down from the midpoint between the bones. Press on the point.

9. Press on the point Gallbladder 39. It is on the outer side of the leg, at four fingers' width above the ankle, between the shinbone and Achilles tendon. The point is very close to the bone, but not on it.

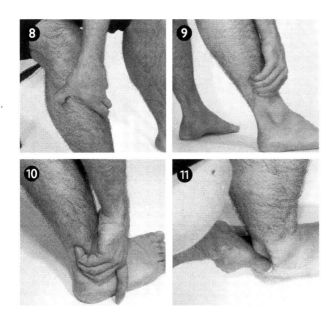

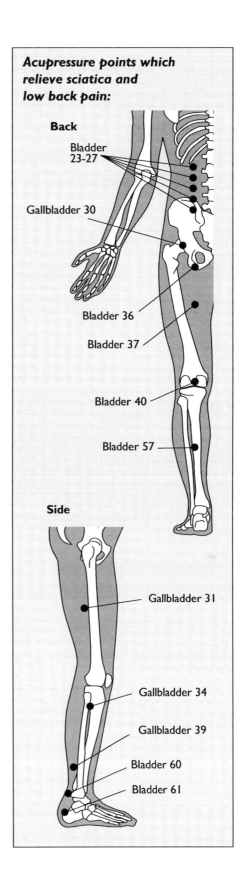

Acupressure points which relieve sciatica and low back pain:

Back

Bladder 23-27

Gallbladder 30

Bladder 36

Bladder 37

Bladder 40

Bladder 57

Side

Gallbladder 31

Gallbladder 34

Gallbladder 39

Bladder 60

Bladder 61

10. Press on the point Bladder 60 on the outer side of the ankle, in the depression between lateral malleolus and Achilles tendon.

11. Press on Bladder 61, which is located on the heel bone, at one thumb's width below the previous point. This point feels tender under pressure.

Follow these steps if you treat someone else.

Ask your partner to lie down on his or her chest. Press first with your thumbs up and down the back muscles on both sides of the spine. Start from the lower back and continue pressing until you are at halfway of the sacrum. Press the lower back very gently and ask your partner to give you feedback about the pressure. Repeat the same three times. Then use the same point combination as described above. When you press on the points in the buttocks and thighs, use your fists and rest your body on the arms.

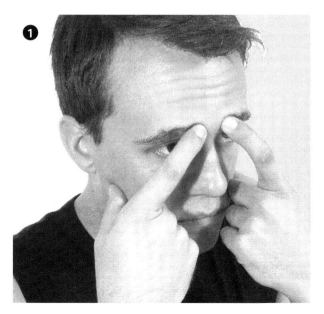 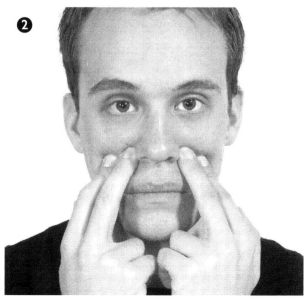

Sinusitis

Acute sinus pain is often caused by a secondary infection following the flu. You can relieve its symptoms, such as congestion and feeling of pressure on the forehead and cheeks, by means of the following treatment. It is important, however, to also consult a medical doctor. Chronic head cold and stuffiness is usually a sign of an allergy to some foods or outside stimulation. Its treatment requires a lot of time and persistence.

Press on the following points several times a day.

1. Place your fingers on the inner or medial extremity of the eyebrow. The point Bladder 2 is located on the upper corner of the eye socket. Press up toward the bone. It is easier to press if you tilt your head down and let it relax onto your forefingers.

2. Place your middle and index fingers beside your nostrils underneath the cheekbones. There you will find the points Large Intestine 20 and Stomach 3. Press up toward the bone.

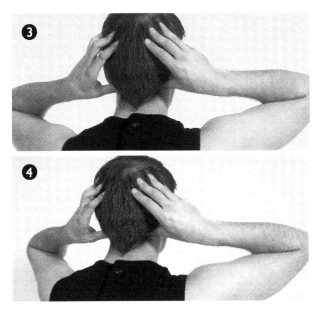

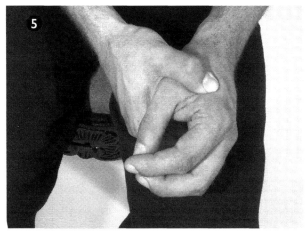

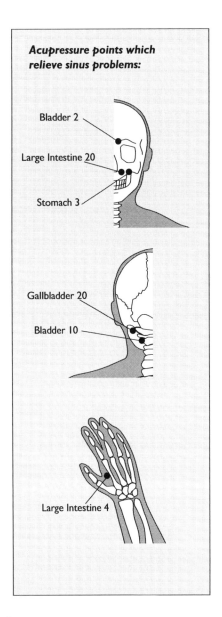

Acupressure points which relieve sinus problems:

Bladder 2

Large Intestine 20

Stomach 3

Gallbladder 20

Bladder 10

Large Intestine 4

3. Place both of your thumbs underneath the base of your skull. The point Gallbladder 20 is located in the depression between the sternocleidomastoideus and trapezius muscles. Tilt your head back to relax on your thumbs and press firmly up toward the bone. Keep the pressure steady, do not massage or rub. If you feel pain radiating to the forehead, keep pressing until the pain disappears.

4. Move your thumbs along the base of the skull closer to the spine, in the middle of the long tight muscle just next to the spine. Here is located the point Bladder 10. It is one thumb's width above the hairline, under the skull bone. Press up toward the skull bone.

5. Press with your thumb in the web on the back of your hand, between the thumb and the forefinger. This point is Large Intestine 4, the best-known point for aches and pain in traditional Chinese medicine. Press toward the bone that connects with your index finger.

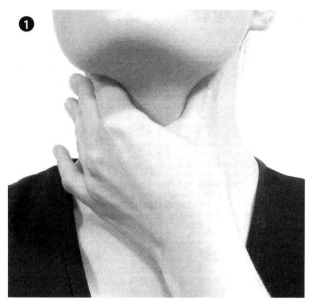 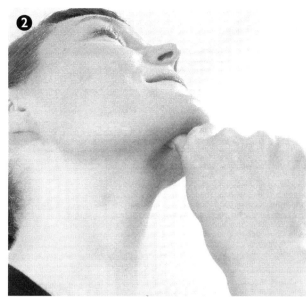

Sore Throat

1. Grab your throat lightly with your hand so that the thumb and the forefinger are placed in the front of the sternocleidomastoid muscle at the level of the jawbone on both sides of the face. Press with your fingers on the point Small Intestine 17.

2. Press with your thumb under the chin, in the middle of the soft muscle. Here is located the point Shanglianquan. Do not press on the bone.

Next press on the inflammation points Large Intestine 4 and 11:

3. Bend your elbow. Press with your thumb at the end of the elbow crease on the outside of your forearm. This is Large Intestine 11. It relieves fever and infection.

4. Press with your thumb in the web on the back of your hand, between the thumb and the forefinger. This point is Large Intestine 4, the best-known point for aches and flu in Chinese Medicine. Press toward the bone that connects with your index finger.

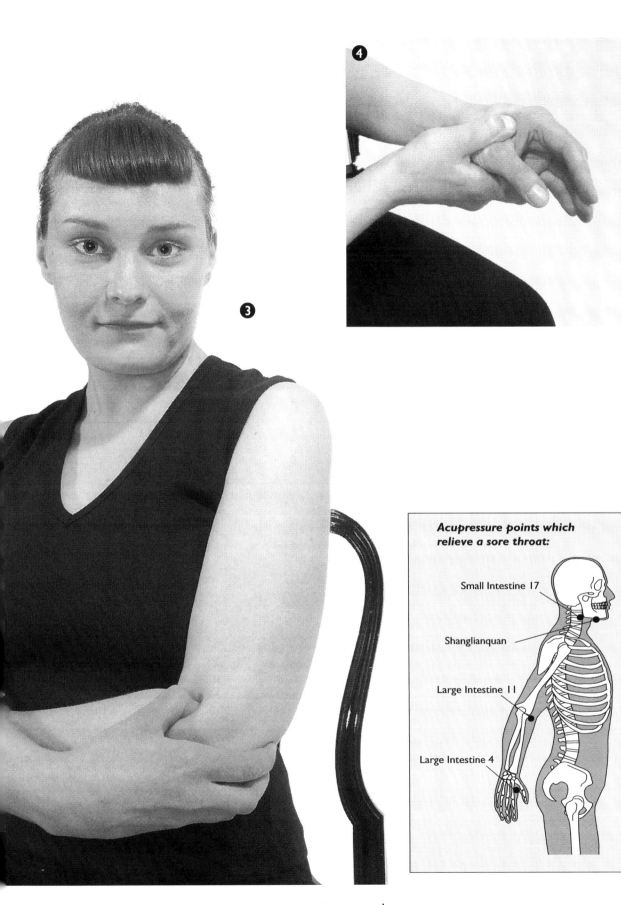

❸

❹

Acupressure points which relieve a sore throat:

Small Intestine 17

Shanglianquan

Large Intestine 11

Large Intestine 4

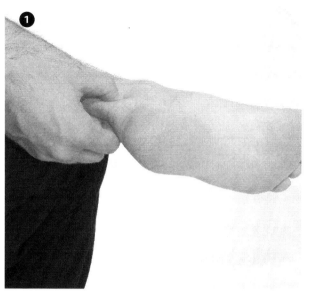 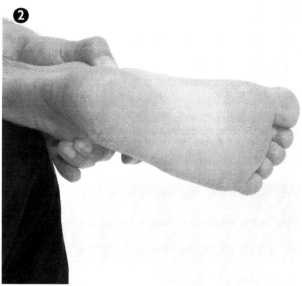

Sprained Ankle

Acupressure strengthens the ankles and helps to relieve the pain and swelling after a sprain. Before the treatment it is beneficial to lift the feet on a chair and slightly rub the feet, ankles and legs in an upward motion, toward the heart. It improves the blood and lymph circulation and diminishes swelling.

Bend your leg and place the foot on the knee of the other leg when pressing on the points.

1. Place your thumb on the point Kidney 3 on the internal side of the ankle, in the hollow between the internal malleolus and the Achilles tendon. Place your forefinger on the point Bladder 60 on the outside of the ankle, in the hollow between the external malleolus and the Achilles tendon. Firmly press both points toward each other for one minute.

2. Place your thumb on Kidney 6 – one thumb width below the internal malleolus – and your forefinger on Bladder 62 – directly below the external malleolus. Firmly press both points toward each other.

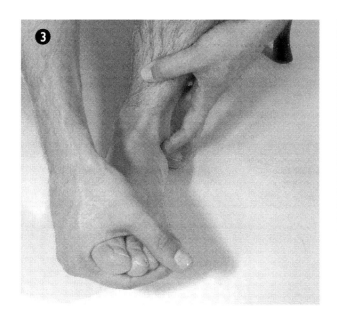

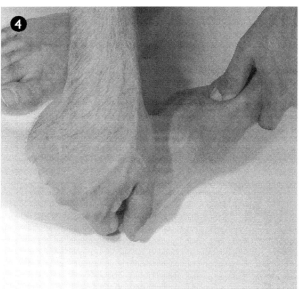

3. Relax your foot. Grab your foot with your hand and turn it outward. A depression is formed on the outside of the ankle bone, in front of the external malleolus. This is Gallbladder 40, an important point to relieve ankle sprain. Press on the point and hold the pressure for one minute.

4. Grab the foot and turn it inward. You'll feel with your finger a small, deep depression on the inside of the ankle, in front of the internal malleolus. This is Spleen 5. Press on the point and hold the pressure for one minute.

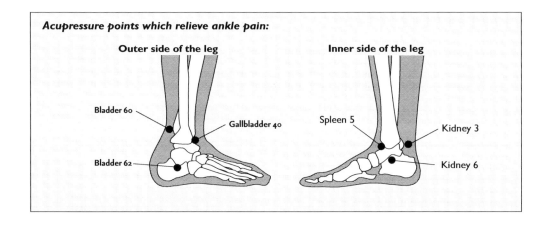

Acupressure points which relieve ankle pain:

Outer side of the leg

Bladder 60
Gallbladder 40
Bladder 62

Inner side of the leg

Spleen 5
Kidney 3
Kidney 6

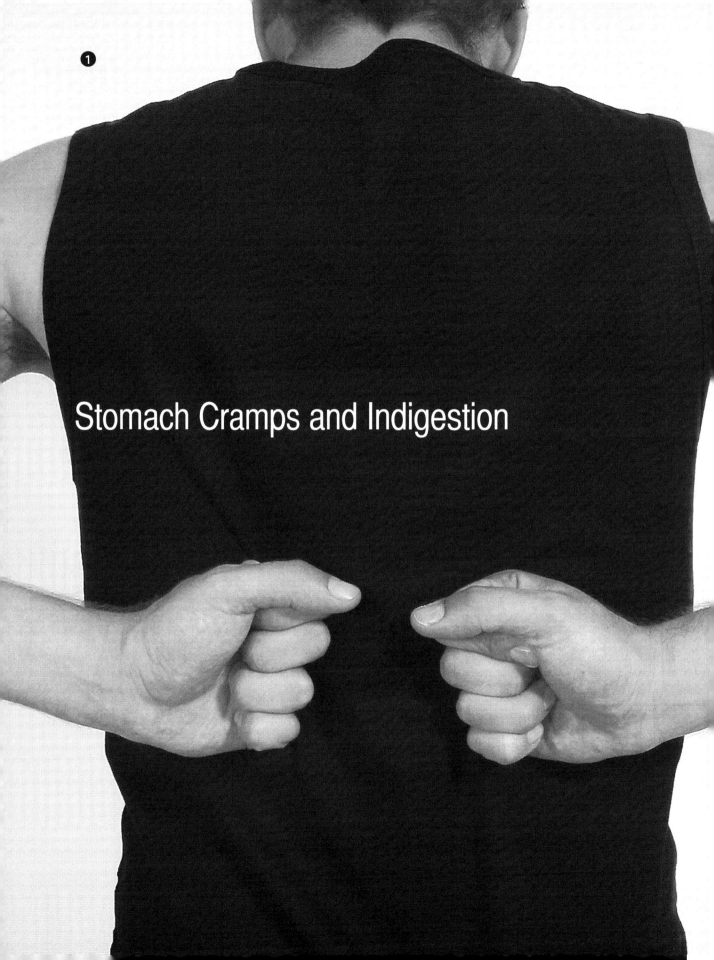

Stomach Cramps and Indigestion

❷

According to traditional Chinese medicine, the digestion is the foundation of the health and wellbeing of a person. Therefore a proper diet and good eating habits are extremely important. It is also advisable to eat always in a calm and restful surrounding and take a rest thereafter. Digestion starts in the mouth; chew the food thoroughly in the mouth before swallowing it and drink only warm liquids while eating. Never fill the stomach totally because overeating drains your energy and makes you tired. The best method to prepare the food is steaming it, which makes the food easy to digest. Always favor local ingredients as they contain more vital energy than ones that have to be transported a long distance.

The Chinese diet is not based on absolute restrictions. The same ingredients might have different effects on different individuals depending on their body and energy types. Illnesses are first treated by food, and medicine is prescribed only if the food does not cure the ailment. "Food is medicine and medicine is food."

1. Rub your back muscles with loose fists below the shoulder blades. You strengthen the important points of liver, gallbladder and pancreas: Bladder 18, 19, 20 and 21. They are located on either side of the spine below the ninth, tenth, eleventh, or twelfth thoracic vertebra.(See example on previous page).

2. Lie down on your back and bend your knees. Place your fingertips or the fist halfway between the base of the breastbone and the belly button. This is Ren 12, an important point for digestion. Press on the point lightly.

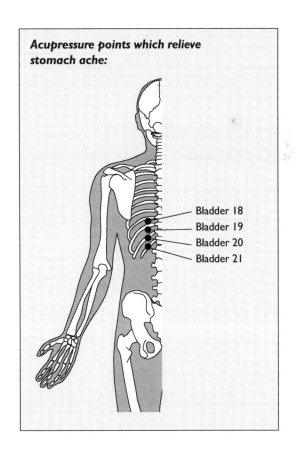

Acupressure points which relieve stomach ache:

— Bladder 18
— Bladder 19
— Bladder 20
— Bladder 21

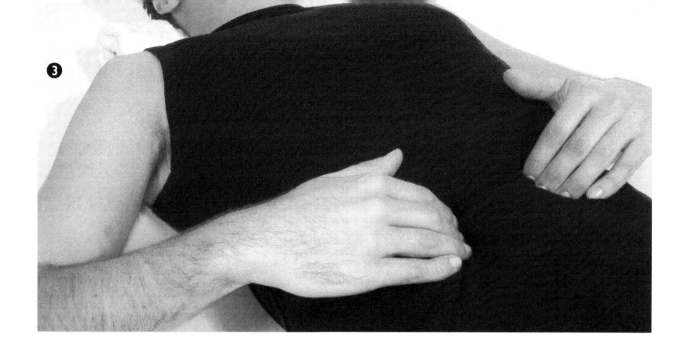

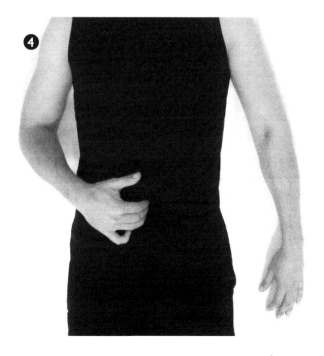

3. Place your hands on both sides of the belly button. The point Stomach 25 is located two fingers' width from the belly button, in the middle of the straight stomach muscle. First press lightly, gradually increasing the depth of the pressure.

4. Place your fingertips four fingers' width below the belly button. This is the point Ren 4. First press lightly, then gradually increase the pressure. Hold the pressure for several minutes and breathe deeply.

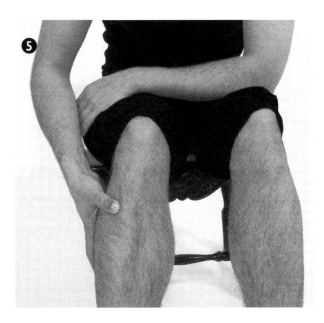

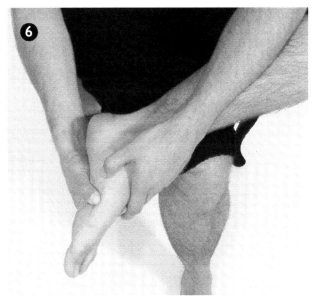

5. Sit on a chair and place your right heel on your left leg. Rub with your heel up and down along the outside of the shinbone. When rubbing the area, you stimulate the Stomach meridian and several digestion points. Press on Stomach 36, which is located four fingers' width below the kneecap, one finger width on the outside or lateral side of the shinbone.

6. Place your thumb in the arch of your foot, one thumb width from the ball of the foot toward the heel. Press on the point Spleen 4.

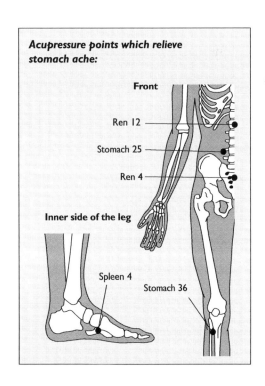

Acupressure points which relieve stomach ache:

Front

Ren 12

Stomach 25

Ren 4

Inner side of the leg

Spleen 4

Stomach 36

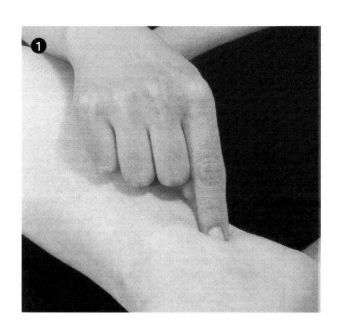

Swelling in the Legs

Acupressure is efficient to relieve water retention which is caused by digestive or hormonal problems. It is also helpful when the swelling is caused by maintaining a standing or sitting position for too long at a time. If the swelling is caused by varicose veins, kidney problems or functional disorders of the heart, it is best to consult a medical doctor to determine the best treatment.

If water retention is in the legs, it is good to raise them to the seat of a chair many times a day. At the same time, stroke the legs with long, light strokes toward the heart to stimulate the blood and lymph circulation.

The following acupressure points relieve and prevent water retention. The treatment should be done several times a day. If the swelling is caused by digestive or hormonal problems, also press some of the points from the chapters on

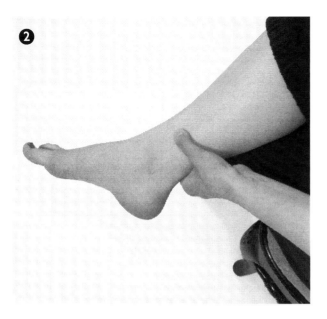

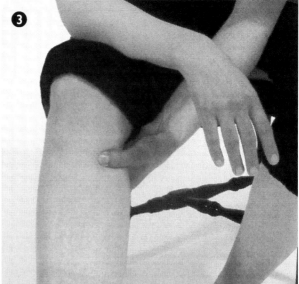

Menstrual Irregularity and Cramps (p. 68) and Stomach Cramps and Indigestion (p. 92).

1. Sit on a chair and press on the point Kidney 3, in the rear part of the inside of the ankle, in the hollow between the internal malleolus and the Achilles tendon.

2. Press on the point Spleen 6. It is located on the inner side of the leg, four fingers' width above the ankle, between the shinbone and Achilles tendon. Find a tender spot in the muscle very close to the bone, but not directly on it.

3. Feel for a big knob below the kneecap, on the inner side of the leg. This is the head of the shinbone. Directly below the head you'll find a very tender area. This is the point Spleen 9. Press on the point.

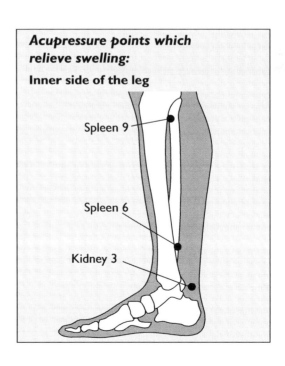

Acupressure points which relieve swelling:

Inner side of the leg

Spleen 9

Spleen 6

Kidney 3

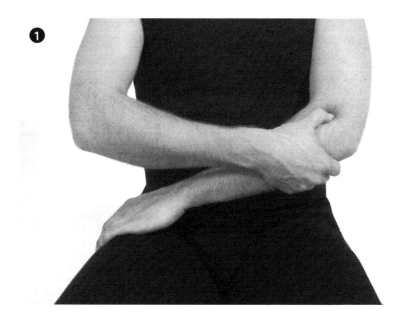

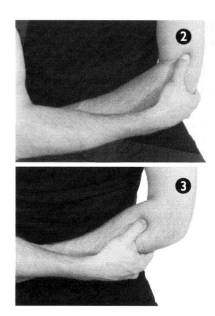

Tennis Elbow

Tennis elbow, inflammation of the elbow joint, is usually caused by overstrain of the muscles in the wrist and fingers. This condition is very painful and it greatly limits the use of the hand as the pain usually radiates from the elbow to the outer side of the forearm. It is, however, better to flex and extend the elbow joint as much as possible.

Acupressure improves the flexibility of the tennis elbow. According to traditional Chinese medicine, most of the acupressure points which relieve tennis elbow are located in the Large Intestine meridian. Therefore, a better bowel function is usually a side effect of this treatment.

1. Bend your elbow. Press with the thumb at the end of the elbow crease on the outside of your forearm. This point is Large Intestine 11. It influences the arms and the elbows and reduces inflammation.

2. Move your finger one thumb width up from the crease along the bone of the upper arm. You will find a very tender spot. This is the point Large Intestine 12. Press toward the bone.

3. With your elbow bent, press on a tender spot about two thumbs' width down from the elbow crease on the thumbs' side of the forearm. This is the point

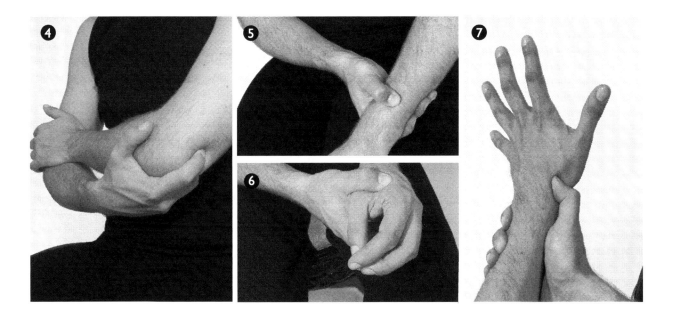

Large Intestine 10. Press on the point firmly against the bone.

4. Place your finger on the back of the upper arm about one thumb width from the elbow. This is the point Triple Warmer 10. Press on the point.

5. Place your thumb on the point Triple Warmer 5 in the middle of the outer side of the forearm, two thumbs' width from the wrist crease. Press on the point firmly.

6. Press with your thumb in the web on the back of your hand, between the thumb and the forefinger. This point is Large Intestine 4, the best-known point for all kinds of aches in traditional Chinese medicine. Press toward the bone that connects with your index finger.

7. Place the thumb of one hand on the outer side of the other hand, at the base of the thumb. Find the point Large Intestine 5 in the following way: Outstretch your palm until a thick tendon becomes apparent on the back of the hand at the base of the thumb. The point Large Intestine 5 is located in the depression on the thumb side of the tendon. Press on the point.

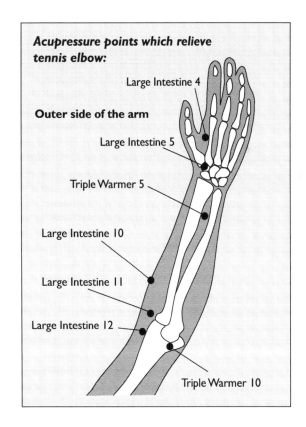

Acupressure points which relieve tennis elbow:

Large Intestine 4

Outer side of the arm

Large Intestine 5

Triple Warmer 5

Large Intestine 10

Large Intestine 11

Large Intestine 12

Triple Warmer 10

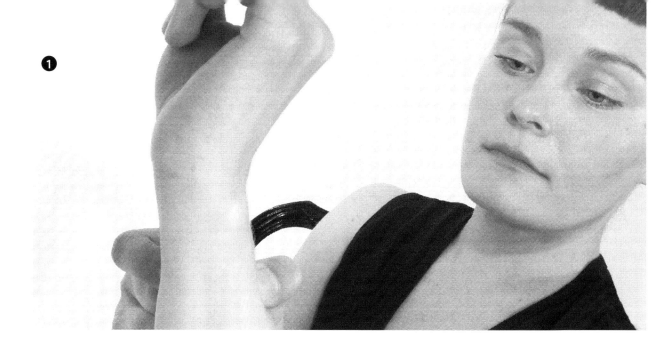

❶

Wrist Pain

Strain, wear, tear, accidents and arthritis can cause the inflammation of the wrist joint. When the wrist is inflamed, it starts swelling, which in turn pinches the nerves. This causes the wrist to start to ache.

Stroke the wrist.
Stroking the wrist daily improves the blood and lymph circulation and relieves inflammation, swelling and numbness of the wrist.

Grab a finger between the thumb and the forefinger of the other hand and stroke it lightly from the tip to the base. Repeat eight times. Go to the next finger until you have done all the fingers. Then stroke the back of the hand from the fingertips to the forearm. Next stroke the arm from fingertips to the shoulder. Repeat eight times.

Press the points:
1. Grab your wrist pressing with the thumb of your left hand on the point Pericardium 6 on your right wrist. It is located in the middle of the inner side of the forearm, two thumbs' width from the wrist crease. Place

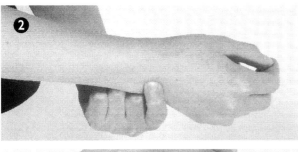

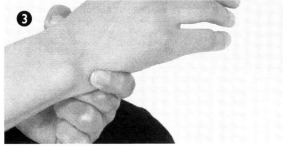

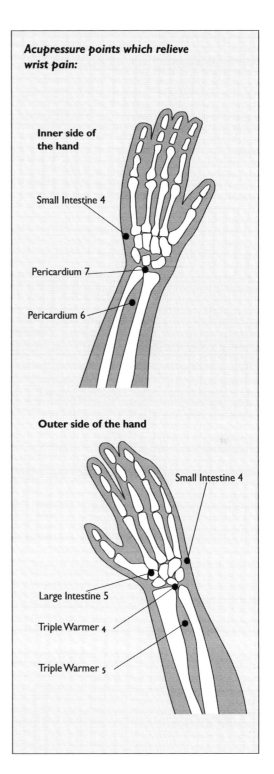

Acupressure points which relieve wrist pain:

Inner side of the hand

Small Intestine 4

Pericardium 7

Pericardium 6

Outer side of the hand

Small Intestine 4

Large Intestine 5

Triple Warmer 4

Triple Warmer 5

your middle finger exactly on the same point on the outer side of the forearm. This point is Triple Warmer 5. Press on the two points firmly toward each other.

2. On the back of the hand in the middle of the wrist crease you will find a depression between the wrist bones. Place your forefinger on the point in the depression on the point Triple Warmer 4.
Place your thumb in the middle of the wrist crease on the opposite side of the hand on the point Pericardium 7. Press on both points firmly toward each other.

3. Place your thumb on the outer side of the hand, at the base of the thumb. On the point Large Intestine 5 find it in the following way: Stretch out your palm until a thick tendon becomes apparent on the back of the hand at the base of the thumb. The point Large Intestine 5 is located in the depression on the side of the tendon that is closer to the base of the palm. Place your middle finger on the opposite side on the wrist joint. Here is located the point Small Intestine 4. Press the two points firmly toward each other.

Special Treatments

Do You Want to Improve Your Love Life?

Acupressure can also improve sexual performance. Thousands of years ago traditional Chinese doctors knew how regular lovemaking can keep a man and woman vigorous and healthy. The curative power of love was therefore a diligently studied branch of Chinese medicine.

The energy that was released during sexual excitement and orgasm was believed to be the basic energy of human beings, which connects us to the energy of the universe. Thus intercourse was a holy experience as well as being healthy.

The famous Yellow Emperor Huang Ti, who lived more than four thousand years ago, was personally interested how sex could be used for the maintenance of optimum health. He ordered his doctors and sexual advisors to write the first manual about the healing power of lovemaking.

According to the book, the man and the woman should spark their sexual desire by playing before sex. This includes massage, fantasies, fragrances, funny sounds, and stories. The goal of lovemaking was not just the orgasm. Every detail from the beginning of foreplay until the end of intercourse should be equally important.

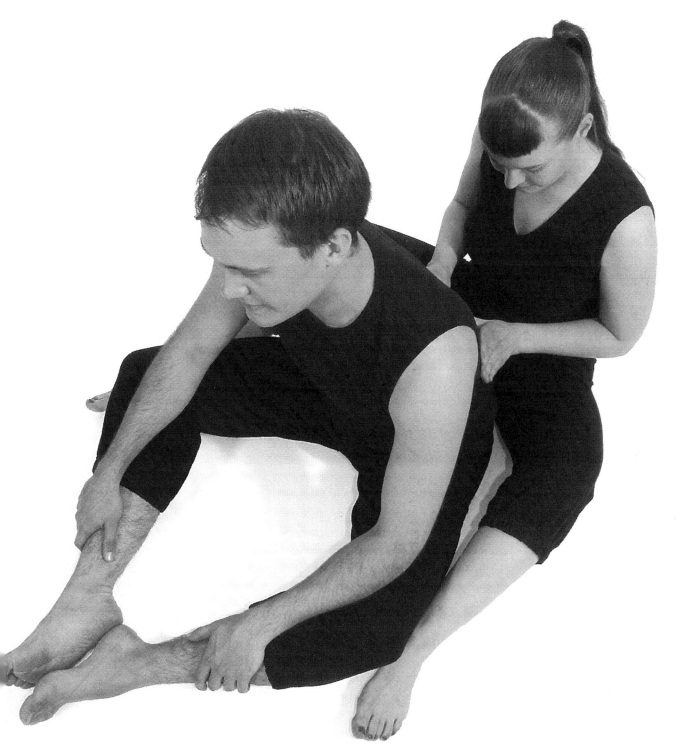

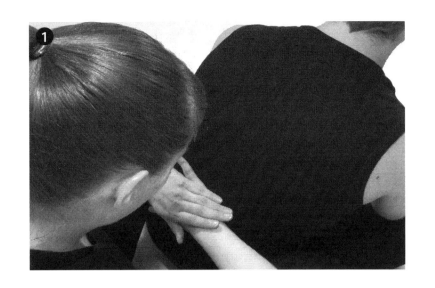

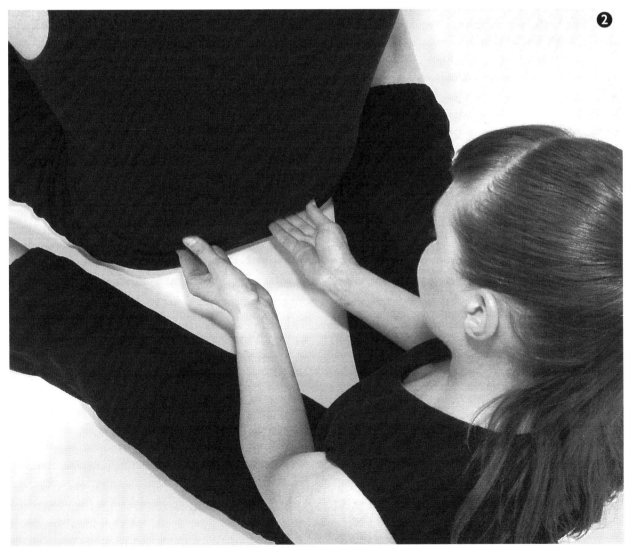

Traditional Chinese doctors pointed out that even if an active sex life is an essential part of health, it can also make a man tired. During the ejaculation he loses some of his vitality with the semen, and that can weaken his immune system. He might even get ill and age before his time. Therefore the man is advised sometimes to restrain himself from ejaculating during intercourse.

The woman can, however, strengthen the man's sexual energy before lovemaking.

Prepare the man before lovemaking:

For sexual energy to circulate freely, you should first relax your partner's back and stomach muscles. On the lower back, one palm width above the waist, you will find the points called "the sea of vitality" and "the gate of life." These points, together with the points in the sacrum, stimulate man's hormonal function. They are used to treat impotence and premature ejaculation.

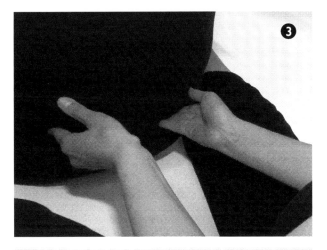

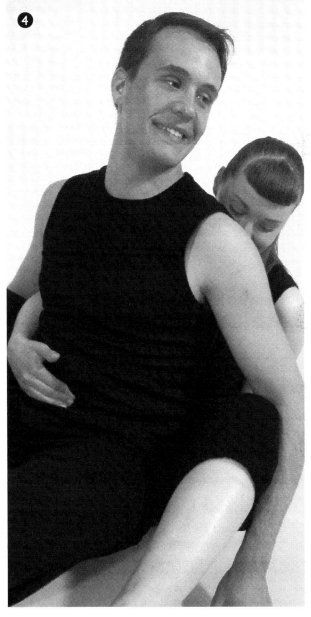

1. Sit down behind your partner so that you are facing his back. First gently touch the tight muscles on both sides of his backbone. Then place your warm hands on the backbone one palm width above the waist. It covers the points Bladder 23 and Du 4. Even a light skin contact produces a sexual energy current.

2. Then press the sacrum below the waist. The points on the sacrum improve his sexual performance. Feel the bone with your fingertips until you find four tiny depressions on both sides of the median line of the sacrum. The points are Bladder 31-34. Press your finger on the depressions or rub them. You stimulate the nerves leading to his genitals. Notice what gives him good sensation and do it.

3. Move your fingers outward from the sacrum and keep on pressing. There are three points in a horizontal line, Bladder 32, 28 and 53 (look at the picture), which helps alleviate impotence. Hold a steady, firm pressure on the points.

4. Continue sitting behind your partner and place your hand on his stomach. Start by pressing on the energy point Ren 6 below the belly bottom. Continue pressing on the median line of the stomach until you come to the point Ren 2, which is above the upper edge of the pubic bone.

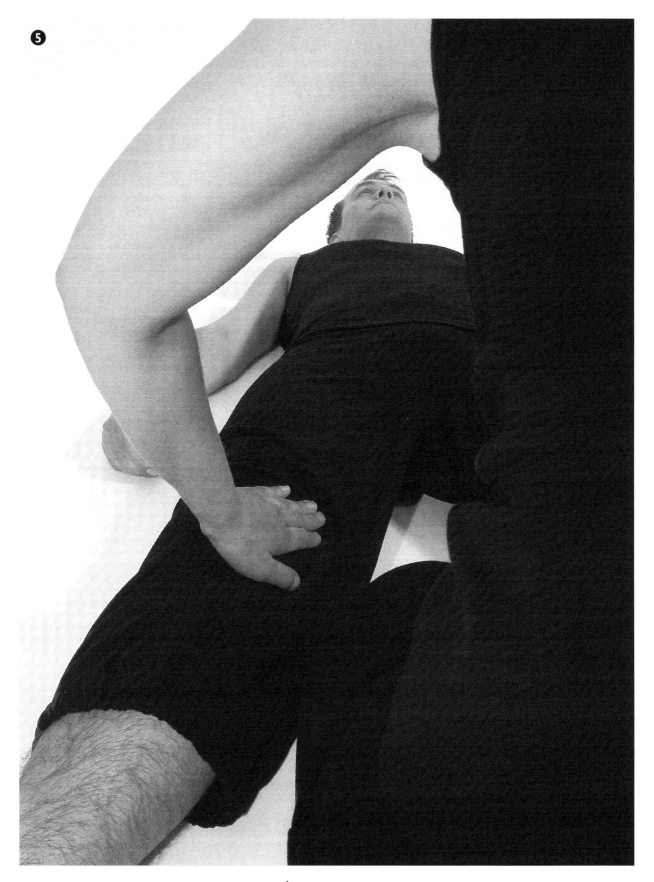

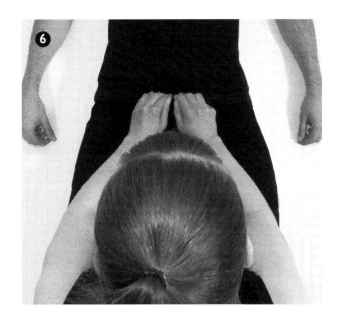

5. Ask your partner to lie down and sit between his legs. Slide your hands slowly on his thighs. Start from the point Liver 9 on the inside of the thigh, about four fingers' width above the knee joint. Press gently with your palms and continue upward. Concentrate on the inner side of the thigh.

6. Place your fingertips above the upper edge of the pubic bone and pull with your hands lightly toward yourself. On the soft muscles just above the bone are located the points Ren 2 and Kidney 11. Press down on the points toward the bone.

7. Place your palms gently on his groin and lean forward. Here are the points Kidney 12 and 13. Press lightly at first and gradually deepen the pressure by using the weight of your own body.

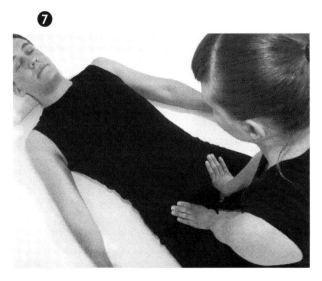

8. Slide your hands under his testicles and stroke the skin lightly. Below the testicles is one of the most important energy points, Ren 1. It is the point of the union of the female and male, Yin and Yang energy.

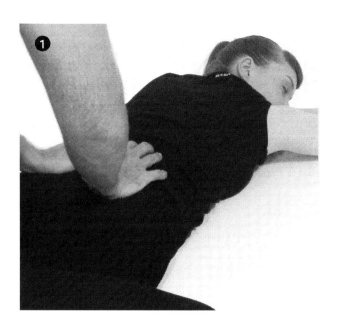

Prepare the woman before lovemaking:

Abundant lovemaking is always beneficial for a woman. She likes slow foreplay with lots of caressing and massage. The touch must be very light and gentle. Use your hands carefully when rubbing her body and pressing the points. Remember that the purpose of this treatment is not to cure an illness but to raise the woman's sexual energy. Massage your partner's whole body before you concentrate on the acupressure points.

1. Ask your partner to lie down on her stomach and stroke her back and neck with oil, using slow movements. Start from the neck and move gradually downward. Rub the back, buttocks, thighs, heels and soles. Then slide your hands back to her sacrum. Feel the bone with your fingers until you find four tiny depressions in a vertical line on both sides of the median line of the bone. These are the points Bladder 31-34. Press or rub the points. Ask your partner for feedback. What feels good?

2. Ask your partner to turn over. Rub oil gently on her arms, fingers, breasts, stomach, thighs, ankles, feet and toes. Place yourself sitting between her legs. Let your hands slide slowly on her thighs. Start from the point Liver 9 on the inside of the thigh, about four fingers' width above the knee joint. Press the point gently with your palms and continue pressing upward. Concentrate on the inner side of the thigh.

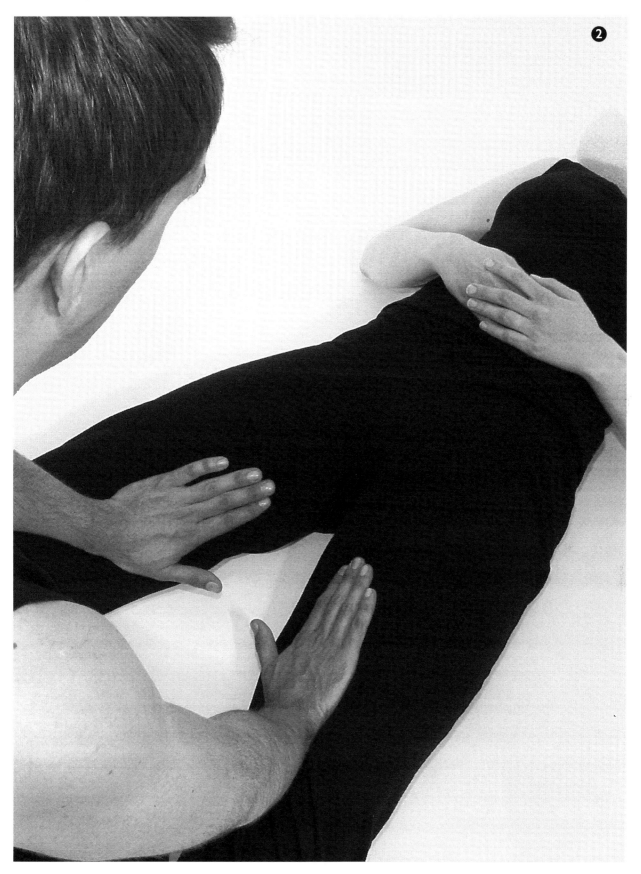

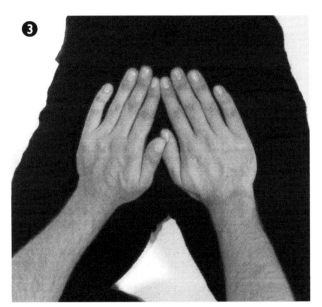

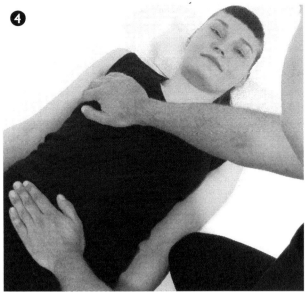

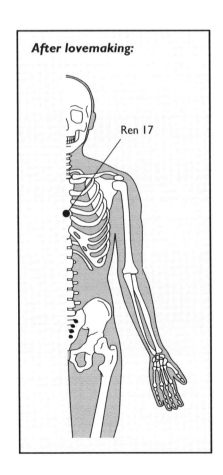

After lovemaking:

Ren 17

3. Place your palms softly on her groin so that your fingers lie on her stomach. On the groin are the points Spleen 12 and 13. Press lightly at first and then gradually deepen the pressure by leaning on your arms. Keep your eyes on her face, so that you do not press too hard.

4. Now place your hand on her stomach. Start by pressing with your hand on the energy point Ren 6 below the belly button. Slide your other hand on her breast, and press her nipple with your fingers. Move to the other breast. The point Stomach 17 is located on the nipple.

5. Place your palms on her pubic bone. On the soft muscles just above the bone are located the points Ren 2 and Kidney 11. Press these points gently.

After lovemaking:
Calm the mind after lovemaking. The point Ren 17 balances the feelings and calms the heart. It is located in the middle of the breastbone, at the level of the nipples. Place your palm there whenever you want to rest or go to sleep with your partner.

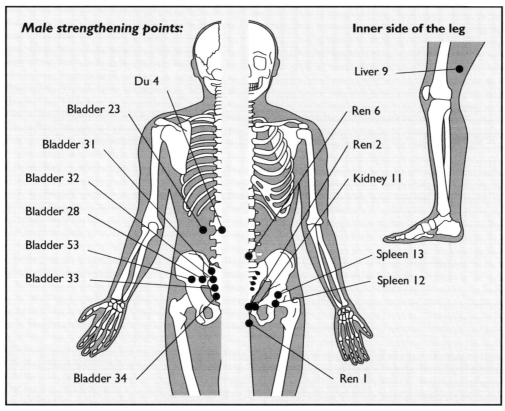

Male strengthening points:

Du 4
Bladder 23
Bladder 31
Bladder 32
Bladder 28
Bladder 53
Bladder 33
Bladder 34

Inner side of the leg

Liver 9
Ren 6
Ren 2
Kidney 11
Spleen 13
Spleen 12
Ren 1

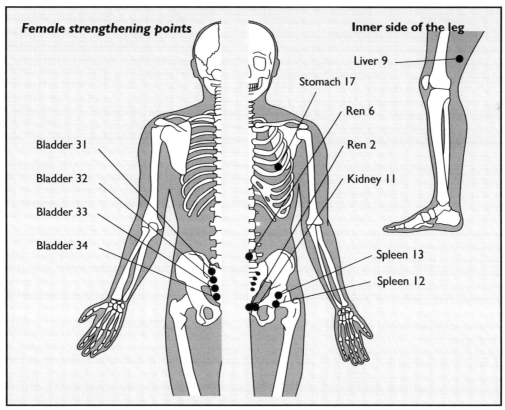

Female strengthening points

Bladder 31
Bladder 32
Bladder 33
Bladder 34

Inner side of the leg

Liver 9
Stomach 17
Ren 6
Ren 2
Kidney 11
Spleen 13
Spleen 12

Chinese Facelift

Our physical and psychological wellbeing is reflected on the face. The face reveals whether we eat healthy food, exercise enough, breathe right, are happy and have peace of mind. Also our bad habits, tension, stress, and lack of sleep put their marks on our faces. Wrinkles, grooves, and swelling start to appear. The skin looks grey and begins to age too soon.

When a traditional Chinese doctor diagnoses an illness, he will first observe the face, namely its expression, color, texture, and muscle tone. According to traditional Chinese medicine the face is crossed by several energy meridians with numerous acupressure points. Muscle tension around the points blocks the energy flow and slows the blood circulation. This hinders cell metabolism and puffy, dry or lifeless areas appear around the points. You can prevent all this by pressing the acupressure points of the face regularly.

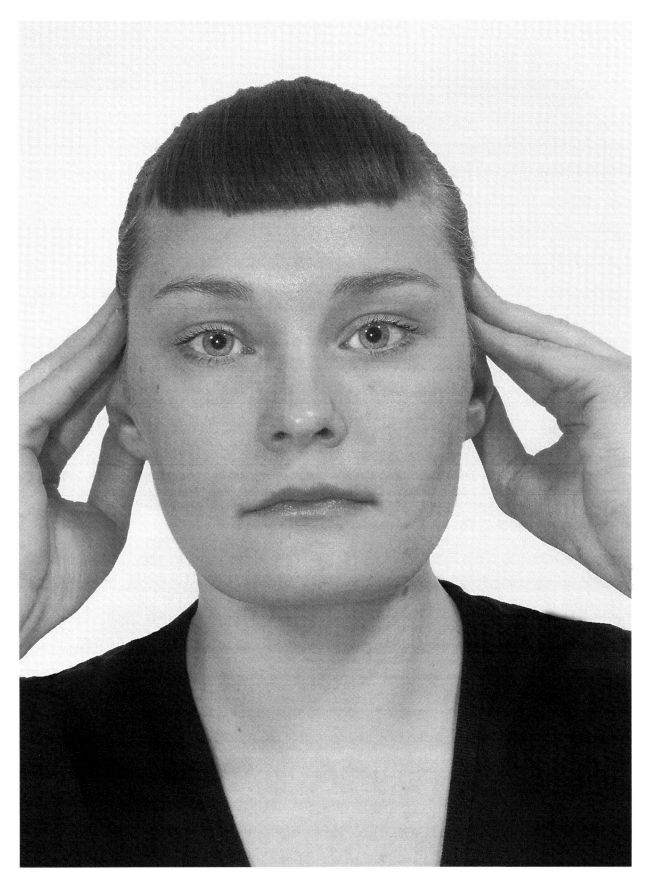

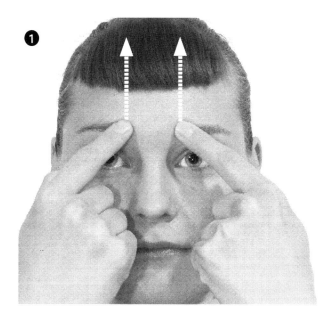

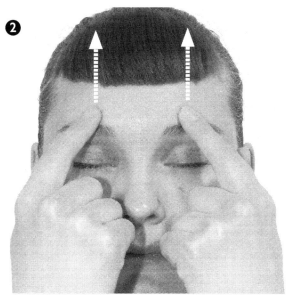

Acupressure relaxes the facial nerves and muscles, so that the tension releases and the energy flows freely. This tones the muscles and stimulates the natural healing forces of the body. The skin begins to look healthier, and the face appears younger. The following treatment is usually done in a Chinese hospital right after acupuncture treatment. It is, however, efficient even without acupuncture.

Here is how to start:

Always wash your hands before you start. Do not use oil or cream on your face during the treament. It only hinders the results.

Do not stretch the skin when you move your finger from one point to another. Press on a point with a finger, hold the pressure for about half a minute, lift the finger from the skin, and move to the next point. Take deep breaths during the treatment. To get the best result you should repeat the face-acupressure twice a day during the first month.

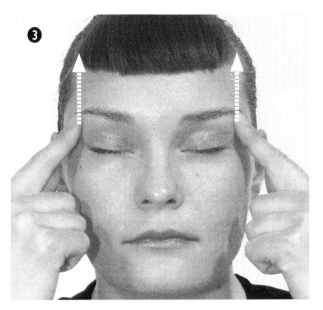

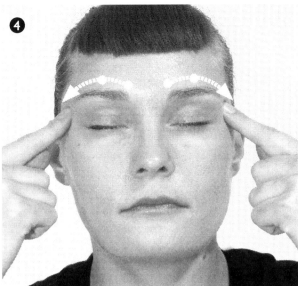

When your face starts to look younger, you can maintain the effect by doing the treatment a couple of times a week.

After the treatment, rub your hands together to create a sensation of heat in your palms. Then close your eyes and place the palms on your face. Take three deep breaths. Finish the treatment by dropping your hands on your lap and relax for a while.

Activate the acupressure points on the face:

(Repeat each pattern three times before you move to the next.)

1. Place your forefingers on the inner or medial extremity of the eyebrows. Start by pressing on the point Bladder 2 on the upper corner of the eye socket. Press up toward the bone. Then move upward toward the hairline, pressing the skin every half an inch with your fingertips, until you have come one inch above the hairline.

2. Next place your fingers directly above the pupils, in the middle of the eyebrow, on the point Yuyao. Start by pressing on the point and move up toward the hairline, pressing the skin with your fingers every half an inch. Directly one thumb width above the middle point of the eyebrow, in a direct vertical line with the pupil, you will find a small depression in the frontal bone. It feels like a tender spot on the bone. This is the point Gallbladder 14. Press on the point longer than the other points and continue up toward the hairline.

3. Start the next line on the outer or lateral extremity of the eyebrows. Press from here upward, like before, until you are above the hairline.

4. Press along the eyebrows: start from the point Bladder 2 in the medial extremity of the eyebrows, continue to Yuyao in the middle of the eyebrows and finish on the point Taiyang on the temples.

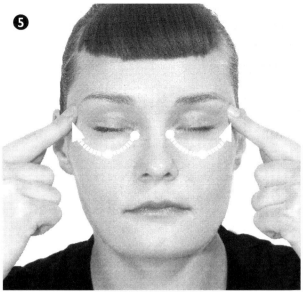

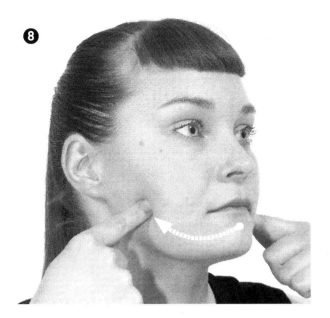

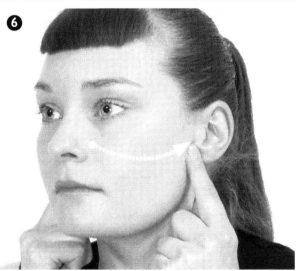

5. Press along the lower edge of the eye socket: start by pressing the point Bladder 1 in the inner corner of the eye. Press on the point very gently. Continue to the point Stomach 2, which is a small depression in the cheekbone just under the pupil. Finish by pressing on Taiyang on the temple.

6. Place your fingers beside the nostrils underneath the cheek-bones. These are the points Large Intestine 20. Press up toward the bone and continue along the cheekbone to the point Stomach 3. It is located below the cheekbone in a direct vertical line with the pupil. Continue pressing until you come to the point Gallbladder 2 in front of the ear, between the jaw and the skull bone.

7. Start from the point Du 26 between the nostrils and the upper lip. Continue until Stomach 4 beside the corner of the mouth. Finish on Stomach 6 in the corner of the jawbone.

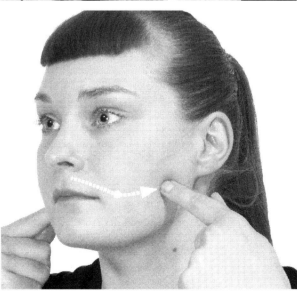

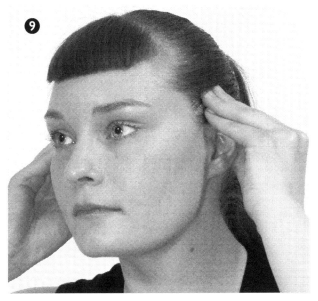

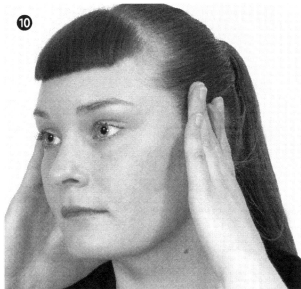

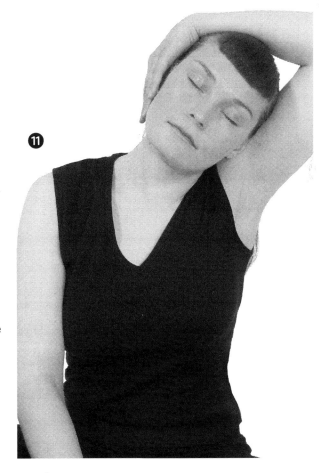

8. Place your finger on the point Ren 24 in the depression between the chin and the lower lip. Press on the point and continue pressing along the jawline until the point Stomach 6 in the corner of the jawbone.

9. Rub your head around the ears. Start at the hairline in front and continue to the base of the skull.

10. Take the earlobes between your fingers and rub them vigorously. There are numerous acupressure points in the earlobe which stimulate the functions of the body.

11. Place your arm around your head and stretch the neck to the side with your arm. Do not bend your head forward but face directly ahead.

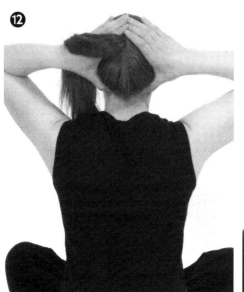

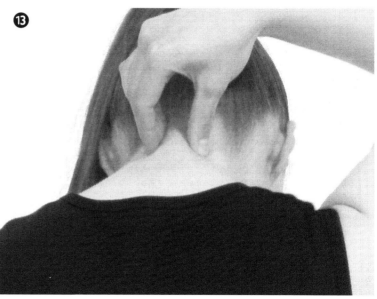

12. Place both of your thumbs underneath the base of your skull. Find the point Gallbladder 20, located in the depression between two big muscles, the sternocleidomastoideus and the trapezius muscles. Tilt your head back to relax on your thumbs and press firmly up toward the bone. Keep the pressure steady: Do not massage or rub.

13. Bend your head forward and stretch your neck. Massage the muscles along the spine.

14. Finish by pulling your hair at the top of your head. You are thus stimulating the point Du 20, which is located in the middle of the crown.

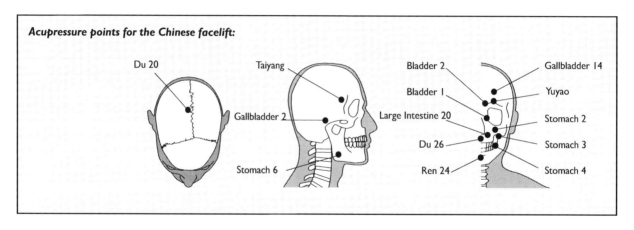

Acupressure points for the Chinese facelift:

Du 20

Taiyang

Gallbladder 2

Stomach 6

Bladder 2

Bladder 1

Large Intestine 20

Du 26

Ren 24

Gallbladder 14

Yuyao

Stomach 2

Stomach 3

Stomach 4

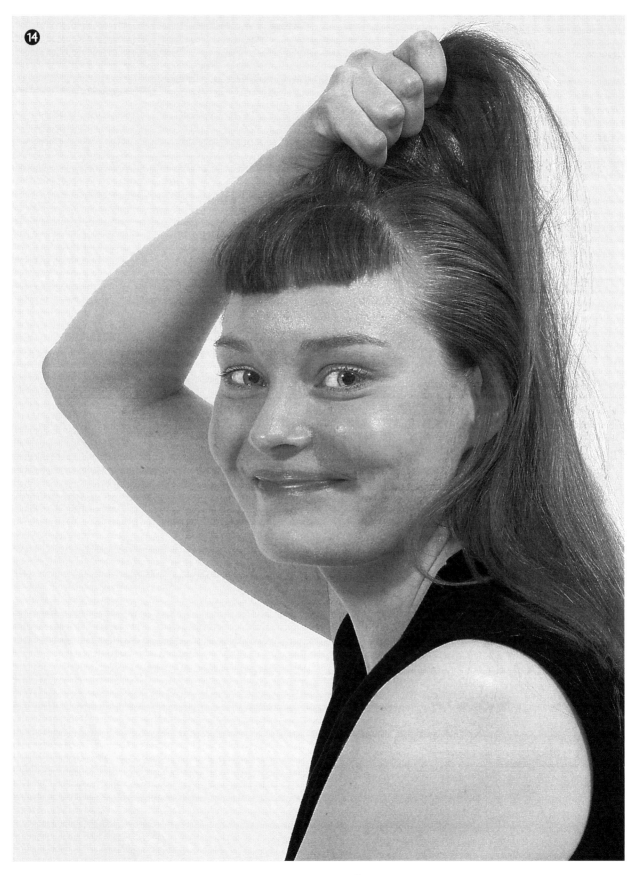

Meridians & Acupressure Points

Daily Flow of Energy

Acupressure points are located in the invisible energy meridians that cross the body like spider webs. They connect with each other and the internal organs and form a uniform energy network. The energy, qi, flows along the meridians. There is a two hour period in every meridian when the energy is at its strongest. This is the daily flow of the energy, used in diagnosing and treating illnesses in traditional Chinese medicine.

If the patient is always waking up at four o'clock in the morning, his lungs might be weak, since four a.m. is the time of the Lung meridian. If he keeps waking up at two a.m., he might have a liver problem, since two a.m. is the time of the Liver meridian. Two a.m. would also be the best time to treat the liver, as it was done in the emperor's court, when traditional Chinese medicine was born.

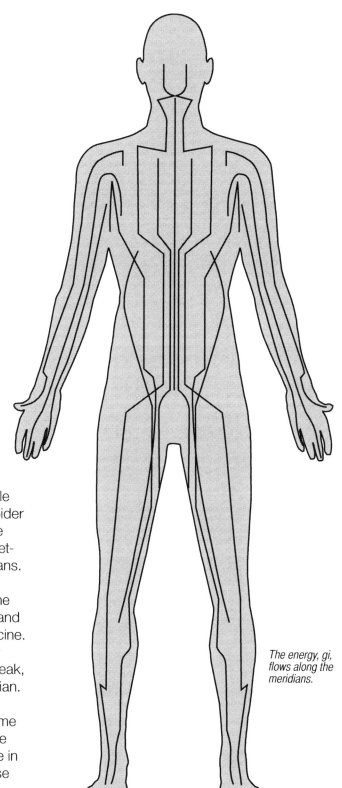

The energy, gi, flows along the meridians.

Daily flow of energy

Time of Day a.m. ⟶   Noon p.m ⟶

	1	2	3	4	5	6	7	8	9	10	11	12	1	2	3	4	5	6	7	8	9	10	11	12
Liver	▓	▓																						
Lung			▓	▓																				
Large Intestine					▓	▓																		
Stomach							▓	▓																
Spleen									▓	▓														
Heart											▓	▓												
Small Intestine													▓	▓										
Bladder															▓	▓								
Kidney																	▓	▓						
Pericardium																			▓	▓				
Triple Warmer																					▓	▓		
Gallbladder																							▓	▓

Meridians, Most Important Points, and Their Indications

In the following list you will see the acupressure points used in this book. They are the most important points from almost five hundred acupressure points known to traditional Chinese medicine.

Remember, there is not one point which would cure an illness alone; several points must be combined depending on the cause of the illness. For example, when treating a headache: first choose the general pain point Large Intestine 4, then add other points depending on whether the headache is caused by neck tension, hormonal problems, stress, insomnia, flu, etc.

In English, the sequence number of the point is added to the abbreviation of the name of the meridian. For example, the first point on the Lung meridian is L1 and the first point on the Large Intestine meridian is LI1.

The original Chinese names of the points are different. They are usually very poetic and tell something about the indication of the point. For example Gallbladder 20 is called Fengchi, Gate of Wind, and Spleen 6 Xuehai, Sea of Blood.

Why is the point in the corner of the eye called Bladder 1, even though it does not treat urination but headaches and eye problems? According to traditional Chinese medicine there is a branch in the Bladder meridian – which runs from the head to the leg – leading to the kidneys and bladder. That's why the English name of the meridian is the Bladder meridian.

Lung Meridian:

Lung 1
cough, asthma, difficulties of breathing, chest pain, pain in the arm

Lung 2
asthma, cough, chest pain, back and shoulder pain, pain in the arm

Lung 5
cough, sore throat, chest pain, pain and swelling of the elbow and arm

Lung 7
headache, migraine, stiff neck, cough, asthma, sore throat, toothache, wrist ache

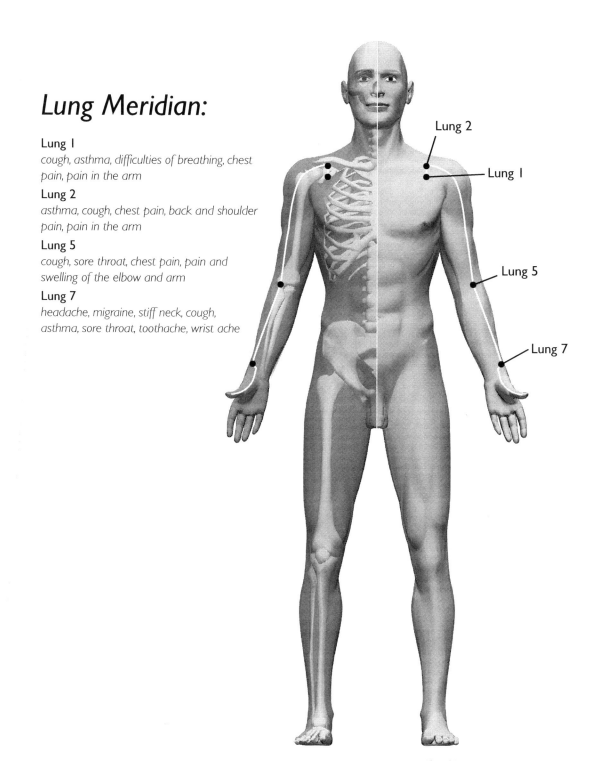

Heart Meridian:

Heart 3
chest pain, stress, tension, numbness of the hand and arm, circulatory disorders

Heart 7
anxiety, insomnia, palpitation, chest pain

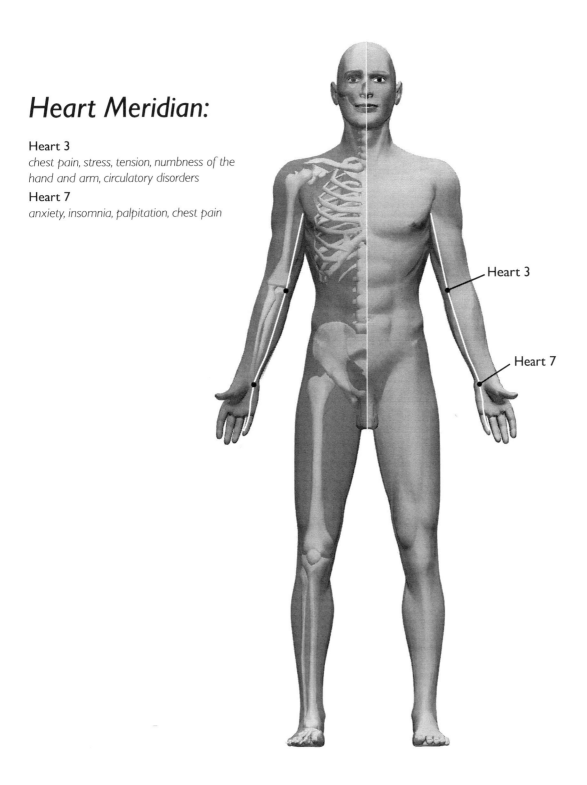

Heart 3

Heart 7

Pericardium Meridian:

Pericardium 4
palpitations, chest pain, numbness of the arms

Pericardium 6
palpitations, stomach ache, nausea, anxiety, nervousness, mental problems, numbness of the arms

Pericardium 7
palpitations, chest pain, stomach ache, nausea, mental problems, insomnia, nervousness

Pericardium 8
palpitations, mental problems, nausea

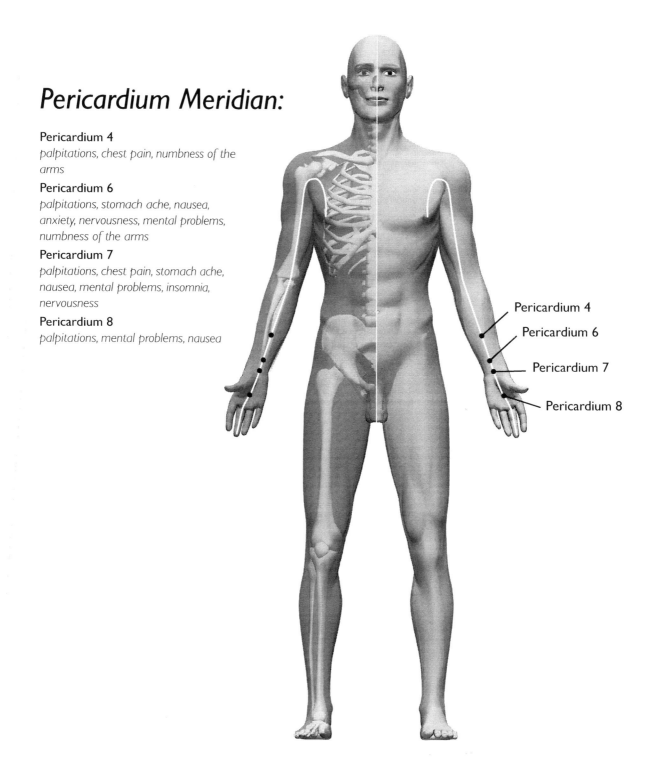

Pericardium 4

Pericardium 6

Pericardium 7

Pericardium 8

Small Intestine Meridian:

Small Intestine 4
headache, pain of the elbow, wrist and finger joints, neck pain

Small Intestine 9
pain in the upper back, shoulders and arm

Small Intestine 10
pain in the shoulder and arm

Small Intestine 11
pain in the shoulder and arm

Small Intestine 12
pain in the shoulder, numbness and aching of the upper extremities

Small Intestine 13
pain in the upper back and shoulder

Small Intestine 14
pain in the upper back and shoulder

Small Intestine 15
pain in the upper back, neck and shoulder, bronchitis, asthma

Small Intestine 17
sore throat, asthma

Small Intestine 19
pain in the ear, ringing in the ears, deafness, toothache

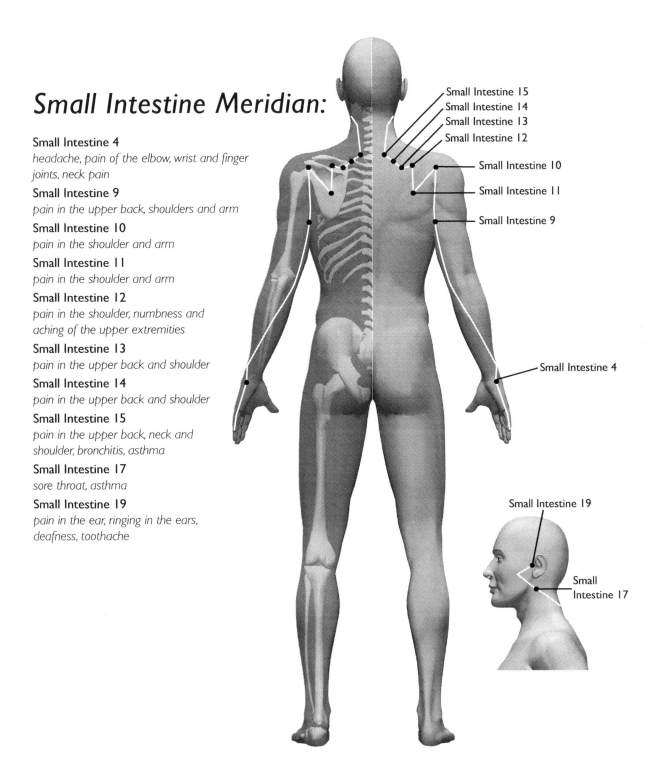

Small Intestine 15
Small Intestine 14
Small Intestine 13
Small Intestine 12
Small Intestine 10
Small Intestine 11
Small Intestine 9
Small Intestine 4
Small Intestine 19
Small Intestine 17

Small Intestine Meridian:

Small Intestine 4
headache, pain of the elbow, wrist and finger joints, neck pain

Small Intestine 9
pain in the upper back, shoulders and arm

Small Intestine 10
pain in the shoulder and arm

Small Intestine 11
pain in the shoulder and arm

Small Intestine 12
pain in the shoulder, numbness and aching of the upper extremities

Small Intestine 13
pain in the upper back and shoulder

Small Intestine 14
pain in the upper back and shoulder

Small Intestine 15
pain in the upper back, neck and shoulder, bronchitis, asthma

Small Intestine 17
sore throat, asthma

Small Intestine 19
pain in the ear, ringing in the ears, deafness, toothache

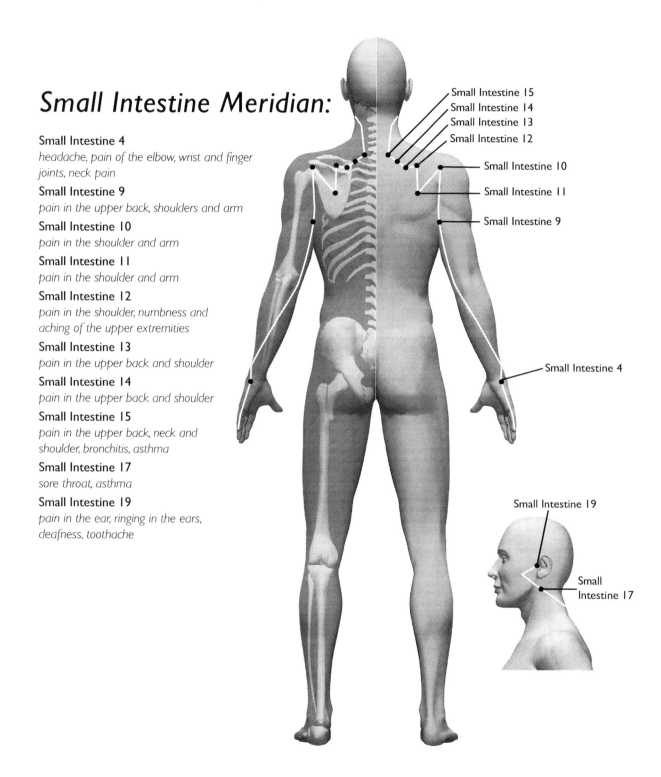

Small Intestine 15
Small Intestine 14
Small Intestine 13
Small Intestine 12
Small Intestine 10
Small Intestine 11
Small Intestine 9
Small Intestine 4
Small Intestine 19
Small Intestine 17

Triple Warmer Meridian:

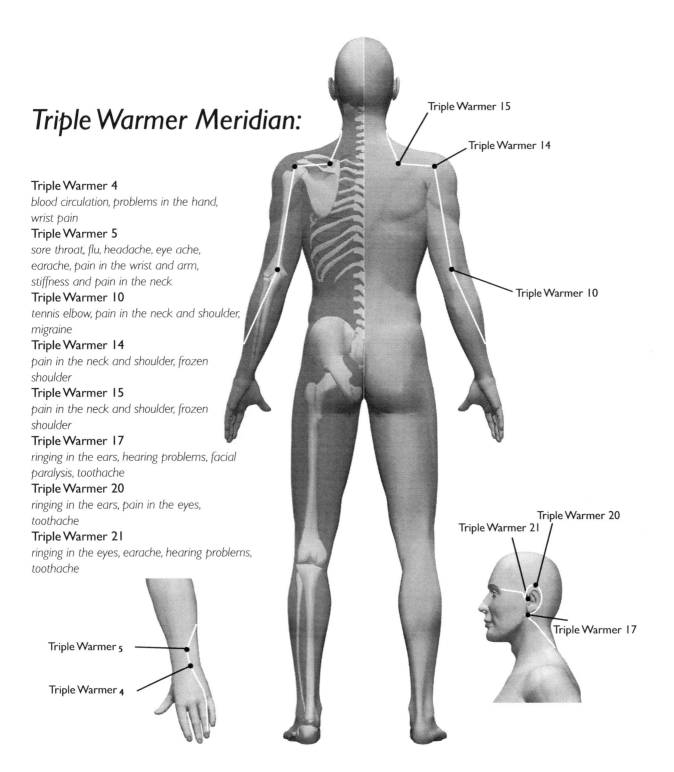

Triple Warmer 4
blood circulation, problems in the hand, wrist pain

Triple Warmer 5
sore throat, flu, headache, eye ache, earache, pain in the wrist and arm, stiffness and pain in the neck

Triple Warmer 10
tennis elbow, pain in the neck and shoulder, migraine

Triple Warmer 14
pain in the neck and shoulder, frozen shoulder

Triple Warmer 15
pain in the neck and shoulder, frozen shoulder

Triple Warmer 17
ringing in the ears, hearing problems, facial paralysis, toothache

Triple Warmer 20
ringing in the ears, pain in the eyes, toothache

Triple Warmer 21
ringing in the eyes, earache, hearing problems, toothache

Triple Warmer 15

Triple Warmer 14

Triple Warmer 10

Triple Warmer 20

Triple Warmer 21

Triple Warmer 17

Triple Warmer 5

Triple Warmer 4

Bladder Meridian:

Bladder 1
headache, pain in the eyes

Bladder 2
headache, pain in the eyes, sinusitis, cold, allergy, facial paralysis

Bladder 10
occipital headache, pain and stiffness in the neck, sore throat, insomnia, shoulder tension

Bladder 13
flu, cough, stiffness in the shoulder

Bladder 14
cough, palpitations, fullness of the chest

Bladder 15
fullness of the chest, palpitations, cough, night sweats

Bladder 18
hepatitis, depression, pain in the lower back

Bladder 19
hepatitis, pain in the lower back

Bladder 20
stomach ache, chronic diarrhea, water retention, nausea, eating disorders, backache

Bladder 23
impotence, nephritis, menstrual and menopausal problems, weakness of the knees, chronic diarrhea, vertigo, ringing in the ears, deafness, water retention, asthma

Bladder 25
pain in the lower back, swelling of the stomach, diarrhea, constipation, sciatica, numbness of the legs

Bladder 27
stomach ache, diarrhea, water retention, incontinence, pain in the lower back, sciatica

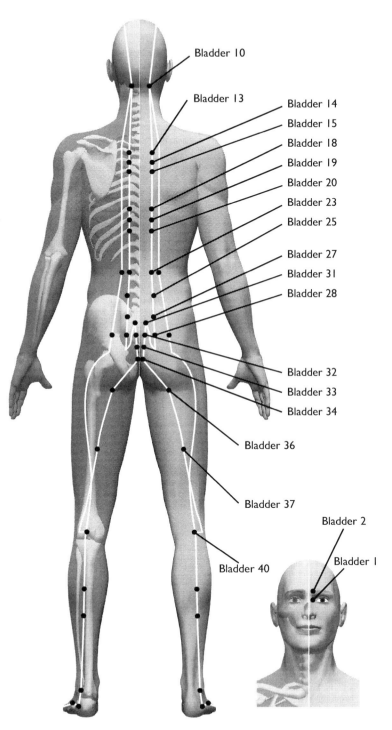

Bladder 10

Bladder 13

Bladder 14
Bladder 15
Bladder 18
Bladder 19
Bladder 20
Bladder 23
Bladder 25
Bladder 27
Bladder 31
Bladder 28

Bladder 32
Bladder 33
Bladder 34

Bladder 36

Bladder 37

Bladder 40

Bladder 2
Bladder 1

Bladder 28

retention of urine, incontinence, diarrhea, constipation, pain in the lower back

Bladder 31 – 34

retention of urine, incontinence, impotence, irregular menstruation

Bladder 36 – 37

sciatica, pain in the lower back, numbness of the legs

Bladder 40

sciatica, pain in the lower back, knee pain, numbness and cramps in the legs, stomach ache, nausea

Bladder 52

impotence, incontinence, menstrual problems, water retention

Bladder 53

water retention, pain in the lower back, incontinence

Bladder 56

sciatica, cramps in the legs, pain in the lower back

Bladder 57

sciatica, cramps in the legs, pain in the lower back

Bladder 60

sciatica, headache, neck and shoulder tension and pain, pain in the heel

Bladder 61

sciatica, pain in the heel

Bladder 62

sciatica, pain in the ankle

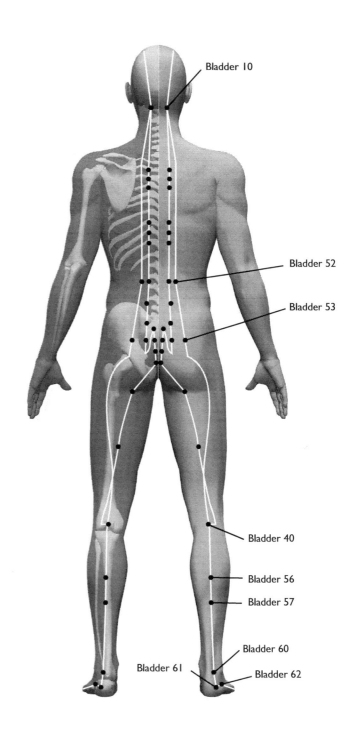

Stomach Meridian:

Stomach 2
inflammation of the eye, facial paralysis, twitching of the eyelids

Stomach 3
stuffiness of the nose, sinusitis, facial paralysis, pain and swelling of the cheek, toothache

Stomach 4
facial paralysis

Stomach 6
grinding the teeth at night, facial paralysis, toothache, swelling of the face

Stomach 25
swelling of the stomach, stomach ache, passing gas, constipation, diarrhea, fluid accumulation

Stomach 29
stomach ache, inguinal hernia, menstrual problems

Stomach 30
inguinal hernia, pain and swelling in the genitals, impotence, menstrual problems

Stomach 34
pain and numbness of the knee, stomach ache

Stomach 35
pain and numbness of the knee

Stomach 36
low immunity, digestive problems, constipation, diarrhea, swelling, general weakness

Stomach 37
stomach ache and swelling, diarrhea, constipation, numbness and paralysis of the leg

Stomach 39
stomach ache, numbness and paralysis of the leg

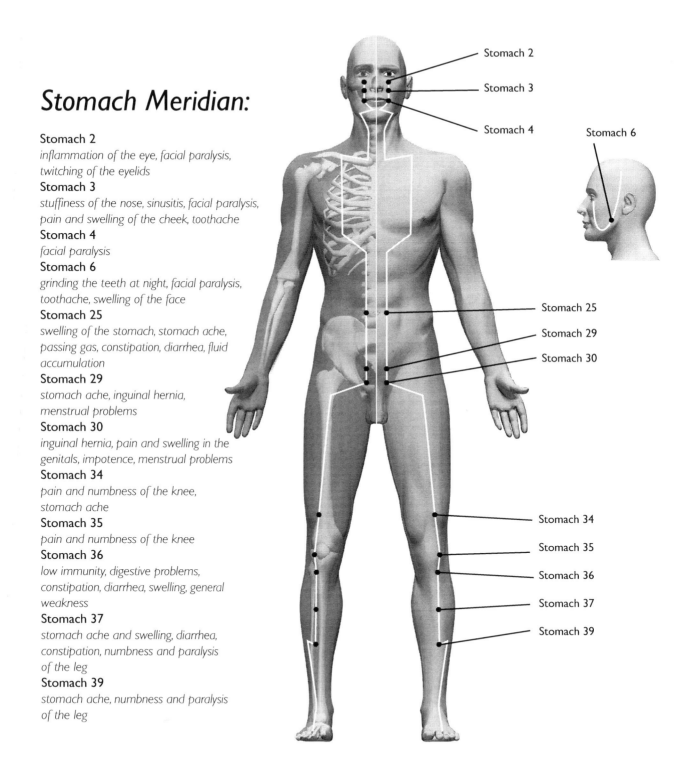

Stomach 2
Stomach 3
Stomach 4
Stomach 6
Stomach 25
Stomach 29
Stomach 30
Stomach 34
Stomach 35
Stomach 36
Stomach 37
Stomach 39

Gallbladder Meridian:

Gallbladder 1
headache, eye problems, facial paralysis
Gallbladder 2
ringing in the ears, earache, facial paralysis
Gallbladder 8
migraine, vertigo
Gallbladder 12
headache, ringing in the ears,
hearing problems
Gallbladder 14
headache, facial paralysis, poor memory,
dizziness, spasm in the eyelids
Gallbladder 20
stress, neck and shoulder tension, sore throat,
headache, flu, dizziness, insomnia
Gallbladder 21
stress, neck and shoulder tension (do not
stimulate during pregnancy)
Gallbladder 30
hip pain, sciatica
Gallbladder 31
sciatica, stiffness in the thigh muscle, hip pain
Gallbladder 34
sciatica, knee pain
Gallbladder 39
sciatica, leg cramp
Gallbladder 40
ankle pain, swelling in the ankles, leg cramp
Gallbladder 41
ankle pain, swelling in the ankles, leg cramp,
head ache, irregular menstruation

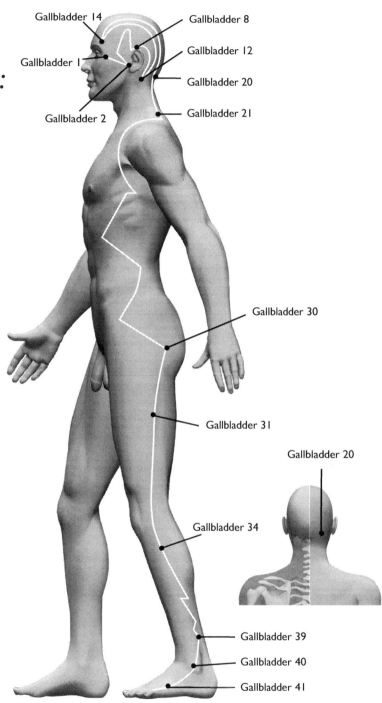

Gallbladder 14
Gallbladder 8
Gallbladder 12
Gallbladder 1
Gallbladder 20
Gallbladder 2
Gallbladder 21
Gallbladder 30
Gallbladder 31
Gallbladder 20
Gallbladder 34
Gallbladder 39
Gallbladder 40
Gallbladder 41

Spleen Meridian:

Spleen 4
digestive problems, stomach ache, nausea, vomiting, diarrhea

Spleen 5
ankle pain

Spleen 6
menstrual pains (do not stimulate during heavy menstrual flow), irregular periods, infertility, impotence, headache, dizziness, insomnia, stomach ache, diarrhea, incontinence

Spleen 9
abdominal distension, water retention, stomach ache, diarrhea, incontinence, irregular periods, pain and numbness of the knee and leg

Spleen 10
irregular menstruation, skin diseases, knee pain

Spleen 12 & 13
hernia, impotence, irregular menstruation

Spleen 15
stomach ache, swelling, diarrhea, constipation

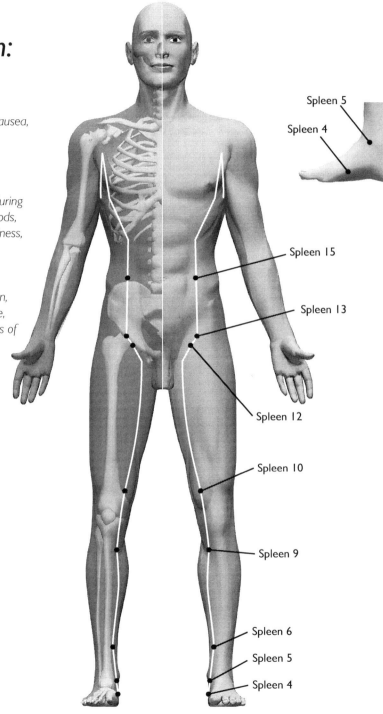

Spleen 5
Spleen 4

Spleen 15
Spleen 13
Spleen 12
Spleen 10
Spleen 9
Spleen 6
Spleen 5
Spleen 4

Kidney Meridian:

Kidney 3
sore throat, toothache, hearing difficulties, earache and ringing in the ears, pain of the lower back, ankle pain, impotence, irregular menstruation, insomnia, incontinence

Kidney 6
insomnia, incontinence, irregular menstruation, sore throat, constipation, ankle pain

Kidney 11
incontinence, impotence

Kidney 12
impotence

Kidney 27
asthma, cough, chest pain

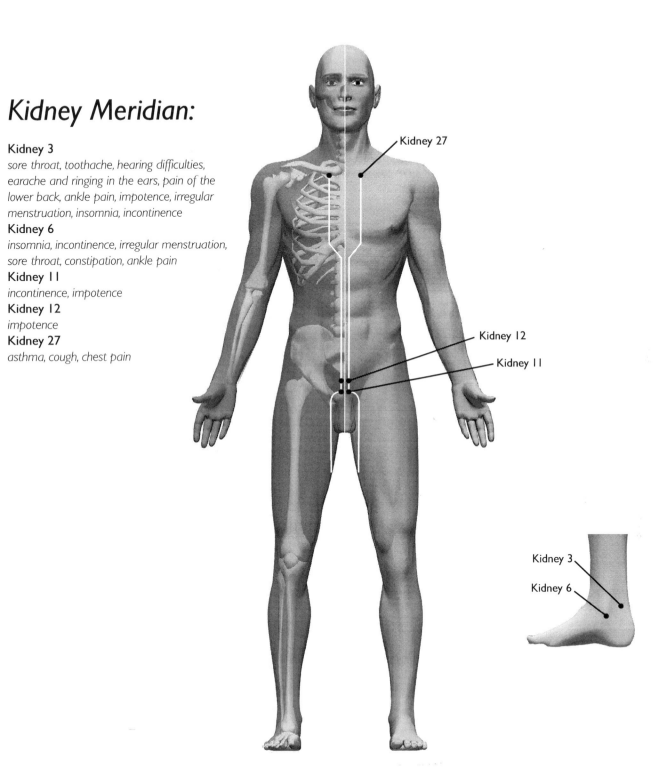

Kidney 27

Kidney 12

Kidney 11

Kidney 3

Kidney 6

Liver Meridian:

Liver 2
irregular menstruation, headache, incontinence

Liver 3
headache, depression, stress, insomnia, cramps in the legs

Liver 8
incontinence, painful periods

Liver 9
irregular menstruation, cramps in the legs, incontinence, pain in the sacrum

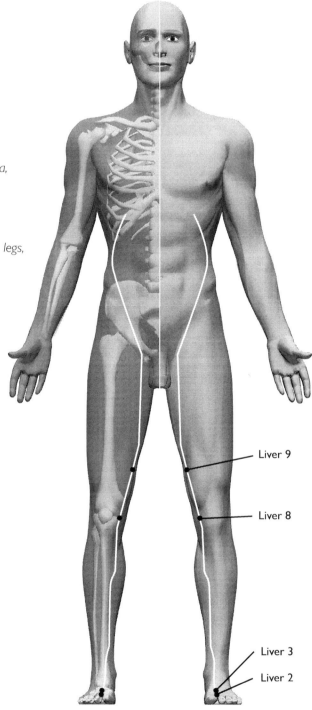

Liver 9

Liver 8

Liver 3

Liver 2

Ren Meridian:

Ren 2–3

problems in urination, impotence, irregular periods

Ren 4

problems in urination, irregular periods, pain in the lower abdomen, digestive problems, diarrhea

Ren 6

stomach ache, impotence, water retention, diarrhea, constipation, menstrual problems

Ren 12

stomach ache, digestive problems, nausea, diarrhea

Ren 17

chest pain, asthma, breathing difficulties, palpitations

Ren 22

asthma, cough, sore throat, horseness

Ren 24

swelling of the face, toothache, facial paralysis

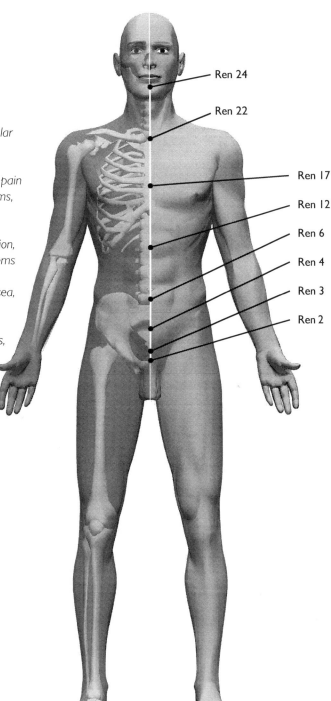

Ren 24
Ren 22
Ren 17
Ren 12
Ren 6
Ren 4
Ren 3
Ren 2

Du Meridian:

Du 4
impotence, menstrual problems

Du 20
headache, vertigo, dizziness, earache, poor memory, stress, tension

Du 26
mental problems, facial paralysis, swelling of the face, unconsiousness

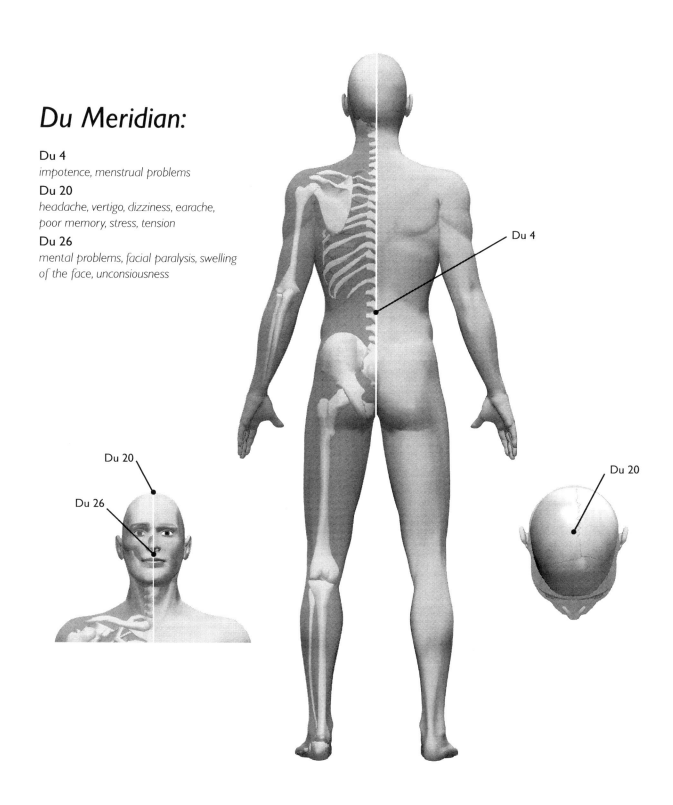

Du 4

Du 20

Du 26

Du 20

Extra Points:

Anmian
insomnia, headache, vertigo

Jianqian
inflammation of the shoulder joint

Heding
knee pain

Shanglianquan
sore throat, hoarseness

Sishencong
headache, poor memory, vertigo, insomnia

Taiyang
headache, pain in the eyes, facial paralysis

Yintang
headache, insomnia, restlessness, nausea in children

Yuyao
swelling and pain in the eyes

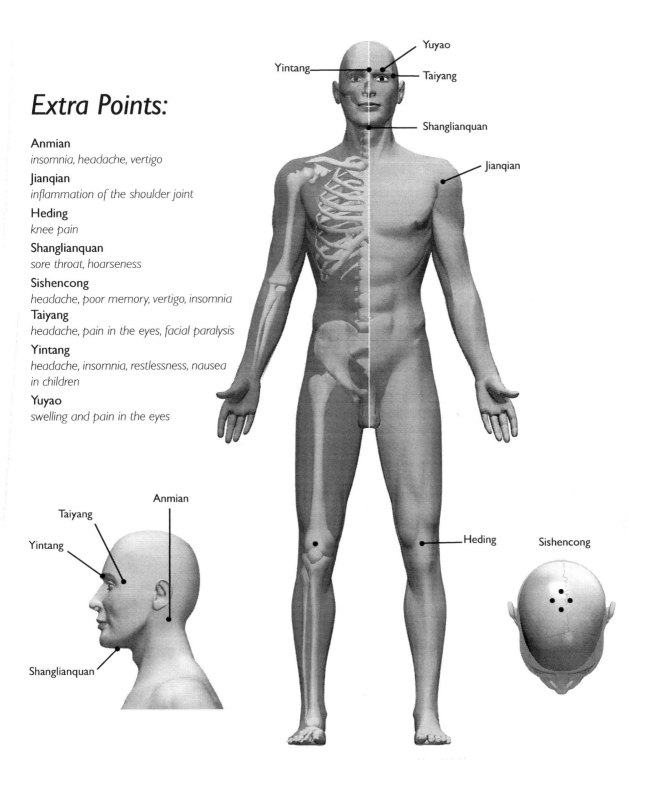

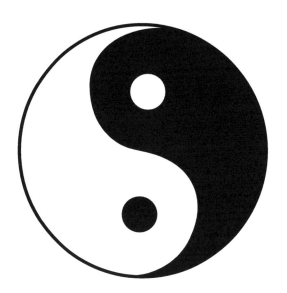

Basic Concepts

According to traditional Chinese medicine, all the properties of the body are either Yin or Yang. The functioning of the whole body is governed by Qi. When Yin, Yang and Qi are in balance, the person is healthy.

Yin is the material foundation of the body, its cells, fluids, and nutrients. Yin supplies fuel for the regeneration of the body. If a person falls ill, his yin starts to diminish, and he must rest to restore it. Yang is the fire of the body. When yang decreases, the metabolism slows down and it must be strengthened by physical exercise. Qi is the energy of the whole body; it is created by food and air. If a person has weak qi, it manifests by tiredness, passivity and weak immunity. Qi can be restored by deep breathing and certain foods.

Differentiation of Syndromes according to Traditional Chinese Medicine

This book uses the classification of illnesses according to Western medicine. The pathology of traditional Chinese medicine would be far too complex to be used in this book. However, a small introduction to the Chinese diagnostics is set forth here.

In the following you will find the symptom groups which are used in traditional Chinese medicine. These symptoms reveal the organ where the problem or the weakness exists. We should, however, remember that even if a person has three symptoms of the heart, it does not mean that he has a heart disease. It simply means that the heart is weak and it might later develop an illness. The goal of the treatment would be to strengthen the heart.

Kidney
Weakness and pain in the lower back, knee pains, ringing in the ears, weak teeth, fear, nightly ejaculations, scanty periods, poor memory, lack of sexual desire, general weakness, low immunity, incontinence, early morning diarrhea.

Liver
Pain under the ribs, bitter taste in the mouth, nausea, depression, irritability, nervousness, menstrual problems, "plum pit in the throat," red eyes and face, headache, nightmares, sleep disturbances, acute ear problems, ringing in the ears, eye problems, brittle nails, dizziness.

Heart
Pale face and tongue, shortness of the breath, palpitations, sweating, pain and stuffiness in the chest, dizziness, insomnia, poor memory, restlessness, anxiety.

Spleen/Pancreas
Tiredness, apathy, pale face, poor appetite, swelling of the stomach after eating, loose stool, diarrhea, constipation, extreme slimness or overweight, lack of appetite in spite of hunger, nausea, vomiting, dry mouth, belching, constant hunger, heartburn, bad breath.

Lungs
Cough, asthma, breathing difficulties, low voice or unwillingness to speak, general weakness, tiredness, paleness, sweating, low immunity, dry or sore throat, hoarseness, flu.

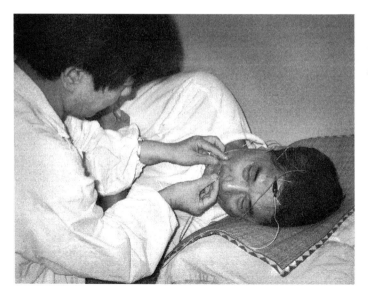

Electricity is often used to stimulate acupressure points.

Notes from the Author

There was a long line of patients sitting on the window side of a narrow corridor. Thin white smoke was rising from their shoulders and elbows.

The corridor was leading to a big treatment room where men, women and children of different ages were lying on tables. Their skin was covered with transparent balls of glass and with needles that were connected to small electronic machines by bright colored electric cords. In the middle of the room stood a wooden cot surrounded by steam.

It was my first day in the Acupuncture Department of the Sixth People's Hospital in Shanghai. I was filled with awe and the place felt somehow ghostly, even though I had studied Oriental Medicine in Los Angeles and worked with Chinese doctors before.

In the corridor was a continuous flow of patients coming and going. They lined themselves up patiently in front of the doctor's desk and waited for their turn, which came whenever a treatment table was free. There were a lot more patients than tables and the staff members were scarce, so the patients helped when they could. One was keeping his eye on the clock, letting the staff know when it was time to take the needles out. Another asked for a seven-star needle and tapped small holes in his own skin with it. This was a preparation for cupping. Many of the patients liked cupping.

Firstly, their skin was tapped vigorously with a seven-star needle, and then a big round glass cup was attached to it. The cup caused local congestion and collected blood from the broken skin.

The smoke that filled the corridor came from burning moxa wool, made from medicinal herbs which were wrapped around the needles. When the wool was ignited, it warmed the needle and caused a mild heat sensation in the surrounding tissue. It was an efficient way to treat a stiff shoulder.

The steam in the room came from a kettle where medicinal herbs were simmering. It was placed under the cot to treat patients who were suffering from back pain.

Those were the treatments we used. They were part of the patients' general treatment plan in the hospital. We also received patients from other departments in the hospital. For diagnosis, our doctor used both traditional Chinese and modern Western Orthodox methods.

Healing Web

My home was in the suburbs of Shanghai, in a tiny flat, sharing a modest cooking and washing area with my neighbors, the Hongyin family. The mother of the family was a high school mathematics teacher, her husband a bookkeeper, and their daughter, 24-year-old Zhao, worked in a Japanese computer company. The whole family lived in a single room with a screen dividing Zhao's desk and bed from the parents.

The Hongyin family was keeping track of my comings and goings, my health, and my daily regime. They sent Zhao every morning to check that I was eating a proper breakfast, and they knocked on my door if they heard me flushing the toilet after hours. I might have fallen sick, they said. I was annoyed at first about their strict way of life, but when I got used to it, I noticed that it gave me a feeling of security and structure to my life.

I stayed healthy in that extremely hot and humid summer of Shanghai.

Daily Rhythm

There are three things that are important in a healthy life, which I learned from the Chinese classics; that life must be a regular flow, with moderation, and it must follow the rhythms of the seasons. The Hongyin family taught me how to live that way.

Zhao came in the evenings to watch television with me. Then her father's voice through the wall: "Zhao, it is ten o'clock." "My father is calling for me, I must go to sleep," she said and vanished quickly to her own side of the wall.

"People here are getting up at six and going to bed at ten," she explained to me later. In order not to disturb my neighbors behind the thin walls, I soon adapted to the same sleeping schedule.

In the hospital I learned about regular eating. "You can go to eat now," my superior told me every day when the clock was twelve o'clock sharp. "When you eat every day exactly at the same time, your stomach starts to get prepared because it knows that it is going to receive food soon. This is good for digestion."

I was later checked that I had eaten a healthy meal in the dining room, and had not just grabbed some sandwiches in the resting area. After the meal was finished it was time for rest, when the whole staff took a nap on the treatment tables.

"Irregularity leads to overfatigue and shortens the life," said doctor Guan Zi in 645 BC. "If a man is sometimes too busy and sometimes too idle, his mind is under too much pressure and his organs get damaged."

In the old times, the day was divided into two-hour periods called Shichens. They emphasized when it was time to massage the body, to eat a bowl of rice, and to take a nap or a quiet walk.

Eat Right

A usual Chinese meal consists of soup, rice, lots of steamed or stir-fried vegetables – raw vegetables are considered harmful – and two kinds of meat in moderate portions. Meat can, however, be replaced by fish or tofu.

The Chinese consume a lot of green tea, which helps digestion, calms the mind and prevents illnesses. They do not like cold drinks, as "a cold drink causes a warm stomach to cramp." On the hottest days, Zhao refused to buy soft drinks, which had been kept in a cooler. She went thirsty instead.

The traditional Chinese diet is a mixture of different tastes and temperatures. There are foods for each of the different seasons. In the morning my neighbors brought me a cup of mung-bean porridge. It is a summer food that lowers the body temperature.

Food is also considered medicine in China. An illness must first be treated with food. Medicine should be used only if food does not bring any results. My neighbors healed my stomach flu with rice wine and red berries.

"The less one eats, the brighter one's mind and longer one's life, the more one eats, the duller one's mind and shorter one's life," says a Chinese classic.

I was recommended to be moderate in eating and to fill my stomach only three-quarters full.

I was told about an American research study where animals were divided into two groups. One was given as much as it wanted while the other went hungry. The hungry animals had a longer life.

Regular Exercise

Light, regular exercise is an important part of the Chinese art of healthy living, because "the running water is never stale and the door-hinge never gets eaten by worms."

The types and forms of exercise, however, are very different from the Western sports. Daoyin, taiji and qigong are the favored Chinese exercises. They are slow, moderate, and best-done outdoors.

Any strenuous exercise can make the body exhausted and sweaty. According to the Chinese medicine, the opening of the sweat glands causes the protective wei-qi to pour out, and the person gets sick more easily.

The flexibility of the joints and the balance of the mind are the goals of Chinese exercise. While strengthening the body is important, one should also learn to concentrate one's mind and circulate the energy. That creates a harmony between a person and his environment.

Because a man is responsible for his own health, he must learn to treat himself. Often at least one member of a Chinese family knows how to use medicinal herbs, and to do massage, cupping, and acupressure.

Patience, balance and joy of life

My teacher, Dr. Huang, told me once that she had been thrown into prison during the Cultural Revolution. "You must have felt very depressed then?" I asked her with compassion. "Depressed? Why? I already was in prison," she answered.

Dr. Huang sat four years behind bars because her fellow doctor was an informant. "Did you press charges against him later?" "I thought about it, but decided not to," she answered. "It would have made working together more difficult."

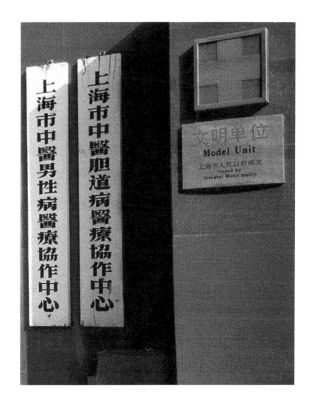

We Westerners do not usually have such patience. I have treated many patients with chronic illnesses, and already after one treatment some of them come to a conclusion that the treatments are of no use.

The healing of the body is slow and gradual. There might be rapid improvement at first, and then nothing seems to happen, until improvement starts again. Sometimes the opposite is the case: at first the treatment seems to make the illness even worse, before the body starts to slowly heal.

Because only very few of us have time and opportunity to go to different treatments for months and years to come, it is important that we learn to treat ourselves. Acupressure is one of the easiest self-help treatment methods. It is also very efficient.

Adriana Germain

Depression seems to be rare in the culture, where the greatest of difficulties are accepted as a part of the normal flow of life. One believes that if man has patience and time to wait long enough, everything will again turn to its opposite.

Despite all the hardships of her life, Dr. Huang was always good-tempered and cheerful. The general atmosphere in the hospital was optimistic, and I never heard anybody complaining.

A Chinese classic says: "If one has few desires, his mind will naturally be peaceful. Just look at the secluded hills and remote valleys. Most people there enjoy long life spans because they have few desires and always remain peaceful in mind."

Patients came to the acupuncture department in the Sixth People's Hospital three times a week, and the treatments were taking, in some cases, weeks, months and sometimes years. The longer the sickness lasted, the longer was the treatment. The drastic measures, like surgery, were used only when all other means had been tried without success.

Bibliography

Gach, Michael Reed: *Acupressure for Lovers:
Secrets of Touch for Increasing Intimacy,*
New York 1997.

Gach, Michael Reed: *Acupressure's Potent Points:
A Guide to Self-Care for Common Ailments,*
New York 1990.

Jwing-Ming, Yang: *Chinese Qigong Massage,*
Massachusetts 1992.

Laitinen, Jaakko & Laitinen, Marjukka: *Akupunktio,
THS,* Helsinki 2001.

Mann, Felix: *Acupuncture: The Ancient Chinese Art
of Healing and How It Works Scientifically,*
New York 1973.

O´Connor, John & Bensky, Dan (edit.): *Acupuncture,
a Comprehensive Text, Shanghai College of
Traditional Medicine,* Chicago 1981.

Serizawa, Katsusuke: *Tsubo: Vital Points for Oriental
Therapy,* New York 1992.

Xinnong, Cheng (edit.): *Chinese Acupuncture and
Moxibustion,* Beijing 1987.

37130475R00083

Printed in Great Britain
by Amazon